Health care is rapid 

tion and treatment modalities have greatly improved the early treatment and prevention of many disease processes.

Understanding the connection between inflammation and chronic disease has become a major focus in both the dental and medical professions. A myriad of studies have found a significant connection between severe gum disease and high-risk factors for cardiovascular disease.

It's All About the Gums, is a well-researched book by Houston periodontist (dental gum specialist) Dr. Hiru Mathur. In it, she explains how the dental profession is at the forefront of combatting the inflammatory response of gum disease. This is one specific area where the consumer can be proactive and potentially reduce the negative effects of a common problem that can be treated easily and before major chronic problems ensue.

– Dr. David Phelps, D.D.S.

I have been in the dental field for over twenty years. There has definitely been a shift from dentists worrying 'only' about plaque and bacteria in the mouth and treating isolated dental issues to fully appreciating the connection of oral health to overall health. For my periodontal patients, inflammation is a commonality across many of the health issues they are dealing with. I'm thankful for this resource to help educate our patients on the importance of reducing systemic inflammation so that we can be better partners in maintaining their overall health.

– Julie C. Swift, DDS, MS
Board Certified Periodontist

My aunt suffered from severe gum disease and we saw Dr. Mathur for treatment. She recommended we obtain a physical along with gum treatment, which led us to find out that my aunt had diabetes. My aunt's physician worked with us on a comprehensive plan to control her diabetes. Dr. Mathur explained that dental health is linked closely to overall body health. *It's All About the Gums* helped us understand, through the use of simple terms, how gums can be an indicator of overall health. This book will help you save your teeth and prevent serious medical issues. I cannot recommend it enough! Such a fantastic new framework to understand how connected our health is to our gum health!

– R. Shekhani

IT'S ALL ABOUT the GUMS

the mouth & body connection

DR. HIRU MATHUR
Board certified Periodontist

Performance Publishing Group
McKinney, TX

ISBN: 978-1-946629-81-4

I dedicate this book to Mom and Dad, who made me the person I am today. To Sumit, my husband, whose unconditional love and support every moment has built a beautiful life together. And lastly, I dedicate this to my wonderful patients, who never cease to inspire me when they dedicate themselves to their health.

CONTENTS

INTRODUCTION

My father's smile is the starting point of many things for me—my inspiration, my career, and in dentistry, my focus on gum disease. So, it seems fitting that this book should start with him too. Like many little girls, I adored my father. He was loving and kind, with a smile that lit up the room and a laugh that was soul deep. However, it was only after I became an adult and started my career that I came to understand the profound impact this loving and kind man, with his friendly smile and generous disposition, would have on my future.

My grandfather passed away when my father was only 16 years old. Left to support his mother and two siblings, my clever father started his own business. He never showed any bitterness about having to grow up too fast and accept so much responsibility at such a young age. Quite the contrary, he threw himself into his work, pulled his family and friends close, and went out of his way to help others.

Despite his outwardly calm and stalwart demeanor, over the years, my father's body began to show the physical results of the extreme stress he had carried since he was a young man. Before he was 30 years old, he developed type 2 diabetes. Just as my father absorbed everyone's problems as his own, so did our family. Throughout my childhood, we never ate sweets at home in order to support my father's efforts to maintain his blood sugar level. However, as all doctors will tell you, diet is only one piece of the puzzle. Continued stress made it difficult for my father to control his diabetes. His health continued to decline, and, as a result, he developed heart disease.

After completing my dental residency in periodontics and starting my practice, I discovered that my father was struggling with serious dental issues. He had advanced periodontal disease; his teeth had shifted and were loose. He was a man who truly enjoyed eating and had many favorite foods, but because chewing was now so painful, he was eating less and losing weight. My good looking, 6'2" towering, larger-than-life father now had a gaunt, aged appearance.

Like they say, what you feel inside eventually makes its way to the outside. He started feeling self-conscious. He had always been outgoing—usually the life of the party—however, the change in his appearance and the pain he was experiencing made him so uncomfortable it started to affect his personality. He did not smile anymore and was very unhappy. His gum disease led to a drastic downward shift in his lifestyle, self-image, and self-worth.

This extreme change in my father opened my eyes to the strong connection between healthy gums and a healthy body and helped me understand how important periodontal treatment is for both physical and psychological well-being.

Once we started managing my father's periodontal disease, he began to better manage his overall health. I say "we" here because an individual suffering from periodontal or gum disease cannot do it by themselves. Recovery and achieving improved health rests on a partnership between patient and doctor. In my father's case, a commitment to regular periodontal checkups opened up a realistic way to fight back. He began to eat better, take daily walks, and he even smiled more. This combination of healthy habits helped my father maintain blood sugar control and fight back periodontal disease throughout the remainder of his life.

Treating my father compelled me to pursue a career as a periodontist and set me on a lifelong quest to help my patients understand the connection between gum disease and their overall health.

Gum disease is occurring at epidemic levels, impacting the lives of millions of people each year. In 2015, a Centers for Disease Control and Prevention (CDC) report published in the *Journal of Periodontology* showed that the prevalence of periodontitis was estimated to be 47.2 percent among American adults (approximately 64.7 million people). For adults age 65 and older, the prevalence jumped to a staggering 70.1 percent. That's 7 in 10 adults over the age of 65 suffering from gum disease, leading to a significant decline in their lifestyle and health! These findings were the result of the most comprehensive periodontal evaluation ever performed in the United States.

It's All About the Gums was born from my father's smile. It outlines a holistic approach to improving well-being through an understanding of gum disease and its profound effects on the rest of the body. It also provides recommendations on achieving health through excellent dental care along with healthy food, regular exercise and medical treatment, for my patients and for everyone else. Statistically speaking, there is a good chance that—whether you know it or not—you or someone you know may have some form of gum disease. I truly hope this book will help you understand the connection between gum disease and other systemic diseases. It provides actionable steps to help you take control of your dental and total body health so you can live your best life.

Chapter 1

INTRODUCTION TO GUM DISEASE

Dentists and dental hygienists around the globe constantly ask their patients the same questions, "How many times a day do you brush your teeth?" and "Do you floss each day?" Since these are often the first questions asked during a dental checkup, it is only fitting that we start here. In my practice, we go even further and ask about diet, exercise habits, and overall health. All these questions may seem a bit intrusive; however, we ask them for a very good reason—we care about our patients.

Everyone knows that brushing and flossing are good for their teeth and gums. What is less understood are the warning signs that our mouths give when we do not properly manage our dental hygiene and how other health conditions can impact, and be impacted by, the health of our teeth and gums.

What Causes Gum Disease?

First, let's clear up a common misconception: just because your teeth and gums do not hurt does not mean your mouth is healthy. Gum disease is a chronic disorder caused by the bacteria in plaque. If left untreated, it will—over time—silently deteriorate the supporting structure of your teeth. Unfortunately, many people do not know they have gum disease until it becomes severe.

In simplest terms, plaque—the sticky residue that collects around the teeth and gum line—contains bacteria. Most people have some plaque buildup off and on over the years because they are not flossing and brushing well enough. Plaque buildup is the body's first signal that your teeth and gums need more attention.

If a person is healthy and maintains good oral hygiene—including daily flossing and brushing a minimum of twice a day—and has regular professional dental cleanings, the plaque will be removed and the bad bacteria controlled. Even if a person skips brushing or flossing occasionally, if they are healthy and have more good bacteria than bad, the good bacteria may be able to fend off the bad bacteria for a while. Some lucky people have enough good bacteria that their bodies can fight the plaque indefinitely. However, for the majority of us, if we stop flossing and brushing our teeth, eventually the plaque will build up so heavily that the bad bacteria will penetrate the gum tissue, and the gums will become swollen, which signals the beginning of gingivitis.

In addition to those who have poor dental hygiene, people who smoke or have health conditions that weaken the immune system also will find an acceleration of gum disease. Of systemic factors, the most concerning are other inflammatory diseases. In these cases, the penetration of bad bacteria inside the gum may overwhelm an already overloaded immune system.

When bacteria attack gum tissue, the immune response causes the body to recruit white blood cells to fight off the bacteria. They are successful if the bacteria are not overloading them. However, if a person has an underlying inflammatory disease and the immune system is overwhelmed, the white blood cells may produce additional inflammation that will then accelerate the deterioration of the gum and bone.

Although we do not fully understand how inflammation in one part of the body impacts inflammation in another part of the body, we do know that the presence of any inflammation plays a role in intensifying the destruction taking place. We also know that the healing process is prolonged unless the patient is taking steps to control their other health conditions. If the patient is receiving treatment and managing their total body health, it can help control their gum disease. Likewise, if the patient's gum disease is controlled, the other health conditions may be easier to control. In this way, we know that there is a correlation between gum health and overall health.

Other factors that may accelerate gum disease are localized and are not impacted by the rest of the body. Localized factors include any areas in the mouth that cause plaque accumulation, including old, broken-down fillings, crowns, crowded or broken teeth, etc. Repairing these plaque-retention areas is another important part of treating gum disease.

Signs and Symptoms of Gum Disease

According to the American Academy of Periodontology, the most common signs of gum disease are:

- Noticeable bleeding when brushing your teeth
- Red, swollen, and tender gums
- Gums that have pulled away from the teeth
- Persistent bad breath
- Gaps between the teeth and gums
- Loose or separating teeth
- A change in the way your teeth fit together when you bite

In more than half of my patients, the first indication that there is something wrong is that they notice bleeding when they brush their teeth. Severe pain is not usually a common early indicator. Gum disease progresses silently, and, many times, gets diagnosed only after it is significantly advanced. In a 1988 study of 1,535 patients, Dr. Claude Nabers found that even though all the patients being studied had advanced periodontitis, 1,371 of them had no tooth loss and were not aware of the extent of damage to the supporting structure of their teeth. If gum disease is left untreated, patients will begin to experience loose teeth, abscesses, and eventually, tooth loss. At that point, there will be severe pain.

Types of Gum Disease

Gingivitis

Gingivitis is the mildest form of gum disease and is identified by swollen gums that bleed easily. The disease is most often a result of inadequate oral hygiene. In 1965, Dr. Harald Loe led a study that showed that if properly treated, gingivitis can be reversed with no permanent damage. Contributing factors of gingivitis are:

- Diabetes
- Smoking
- Stress
- Genetics
- Puberty
- Poor nutrition
- Hormonal changes

- Pregnancy
- Substance abuse
- HIV infection
- Medications

Periodontitis/Periodontal (gum) disease

Untreated gingivitis usually progresses to periodontitis. When plaque builds up so heavily around the teeth that it spreads below the gum line, toxins produced by the bad bacteria irritate the gums. The toxins inflame the gums, and the tissue and bone that support the teeth begin to recede and break down, which is the onset of periodontitis.

According to the original classification, there are four types of periodontitis:

1. **Aggressive form** – This occurs in otherwise healthy individuals and causes rapid tissue and bone loss.
2. **Chronic form** – A very common form of periodontitis that causes inflammation of the supporting tissues of the teeth. Chronic periodontitis is usually found in adults but can occur at any age. The disease progresses slowly but can have periods of rapid progression.
3. **Periodontitis as a manifestation of systemic disease** – This form of periodontitis can occur at any age and is usually associated with a systemic disease such as diabetes, heart disease, etc.

4. **Necrotizing periodontitis** – This form of the disease results in necrosis of tissue and bone and is usually seen in patients with HIV, malnutrition, or immunosuppression.

New classification of periodontitis:

A newer classification of periodontal disease was introduced in 2017 by the American Academy of Periodontology. It includes all diseased conditions, especially the ones affected by systemic disease, thus stressing the importance of this connection. They can be broadly described in these main categories:

1. Periodontal health, gingival health and conditions, which includes healthy conditions, gingivitis caused by plaque and gingival inflammation caused by any other reasons like immune problems, allergies, etc.
2. Periodontitis, which can be caused by bacterial infection that extends into the bone and supporting structures of the tooth due to poor oral hygiene, or it can be a manifestation of some underlying disease.
3. Other conditions that affect the gums and the supporting tooth structures, like leukemia, etc.
4. Inflammation and disease of dental implants.

The table below represents more details of this classification:

Classification of periodontal, peri-implant diseases and conditions, 2017		
Periodontal diseases and conditions		
Periodontal health, gingival diseases and conditions	**Periodontitis**	**Other conditions affecting the periodontium**
Periodontal and gingival health	Necrotizing periodontal disease	Systemic diseas-es, abscesses
Gingivitis biofilm induced	Periodontitis	Traumatic occlusion
Gingival diseases non-dental biofilm induced	Periodontitis as a manifestation of systemic diseases	Mucogingival deformities
Peri-implant diseases and conditions		
Peri-implant health	Peri-implant mucositis, peri-implantitis	Peri-implant tissue deficiencies

As periodontitis progresses into the gum, aggressive bacteria reach deep inside the teeth, down to the root. The periodontal ligaments, which are made of collagen fibers that connect the teeth to the bone and support the teeth, begin to break down. As the toxins stimulate additional chronic inflammation, the bacteria go deeper into the tissue and the supporting bone begins to recede and deteriorate. The gums separate from the teeth, forming deep spaces between the teeth and gums. These spaces, or pockets, then become infected. At this stage of periodontitis, the patient may still feel only minor discomfort.

When the bacteria enter the tissues and bone, they cause a response in the body. The body recognizes the bacteria as foreign agents and starts an inflammatory response by white blood cells. The blood cells produce chemicals to kill the bacteria, but if the inflammation persists, they also produce toxins that activate bone-dissolving cells. These toxins—including collagenase, which is particularly destructive—cause collateral damage and start destroying the collagen in the gum and bone.

As gum disease advances, the onslaught of aggressive bacteria, collagenase, and other toxins wreaks havoc on the tissue and bone. Abscesses form, and the gums bleed during flossing and brushing. Since all the attachments are gone, the gums move away from the teeth, and the pockets become deeper. The teeth begin to shift, and the bone continues to deteriorate.

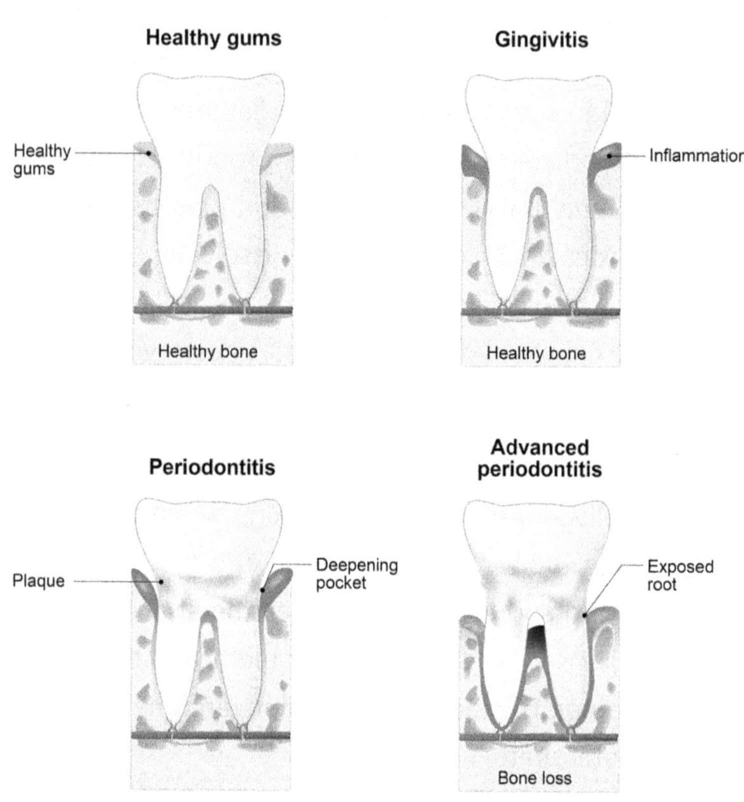

Credit: designiua 123rF.com

The figure above represents the different stages of periodontal disease.

Even if the person was healthy when their gum disease began, by the time they reach this stage of periodontitis, their teeth will be loose, and they will soon begin to feel pain with every bite they eat because they are putting pressure on the deeper tissues.

Treatment of Gum Disease

The initial stage of gum disease, commonly known as gingivitis, is usually reversible in an otherwise healthy person because the disease is still superficial. It is only in the gums and has not penetrated the deeper tissues. At this point, if the patient receives a professional dental cleaning, has any plaque retention areas repaired, begins flossing daily, and brushes their teeth a minimum of twice a day, the disease will go away and leave no permanent damage. As long as the patient continues regular dental checkups and maintains good oral hygiene and good overall health, the disease will not reoccur.

> *This is Susan's case. A young woman in her 30s, Susan came to my practice after visiting an orthodontist. She felt that her teeth were shifting and thought she might need braces. She also told us that her gums were bleeding when she brushed her teeth. Unfortunately, if the disease progresses to bone loss, known as periodontitis, it is chronic and irreversible. As standard practice, the orthodontist referred her to us to diagnose any potential problems before prescribing braces.*
>
> *Most gum disease patients are in their 40s or older, but, as Susan's case shows, periodontal disease can*

advance in younger patients as well due to neglect and plaque retentive areas. We performed a full examination on Susan, which included checking for signs of cancer and TMJ issues, taking x-rays, and measuring her gum pockets to look for evidence of bone loss.

The examination showed that Susan had advanced periodontal disease with a significant amount of bone loss under her molars. She was not experiencing any pain and was completely surprised by the diagnosis. To better understand what had led to the problems, we asked about her overall health and dental hygiene habits.

Susan had smoked during college but was no longer a smoker. She had no underlying health issues and was unaware of any genetic factors that might impact her teeth. However, she told us that she had never been to a dentist, and she had never flossed. She did not know how to properly maintain her dental health. As a consequence, she had developed tiny cavities in between her teeth. The cavities became heavy plaque-retention areas, accelerating the inflammation and bone loss.

Another problem impacting Susan's teeth was that as a child she'd had some teeth extracted that had never been replaced. So, her teeth had shifted and were tilting into the open space and crowding in the front of her mouth, causing heavier plaque collection and inflammation.

Many adults who have molars extracted as children or teenagers do not replace them with dental implants or other replacements and experience shifting teeth in adulthood. If you combine this with periodontal disease and bone loss, the teeth shift even more. Once the teeth start shifting, they collect more plaque, which leads to more inflammation and bone loss. Susan was stuck in this vicious cycle.

Treatment for periodontitis focuses on controlling the impact of the disease to prevent further damage to the gums, bone, and teeth. Most people will not feel severe pain until the disease is quite advanced, which is why gum disease can progress unchecked for a long time. So, an otherwise healthy person may not feel any pain, but they may notice that their teeth have shifted. I frequently encounter patients in this situation who come to my practice in an attempt to figure out what is happening.

Periodontists are dental specialists who go through additional training after dental school to mainly focus on treating periodontal disease with surgical and non-surgical methods. They also place dental implants in the bone to replace missing teeth. Periodontists or their hygienists work to remove all the bacteria, which can be done with deep cleaning or scaling and root planing after numbing the affected areas and removing the adherent bacteria from the root surfaces. If this does not resolve the infection then periodontists are involved in treating the deeper areas by accessing them with gum surgery. Gum surgery may be performed by numbing the affected areas with or without sedation, using traditional scalpels or lasers to reach the deep, infected areas to clean out the infection and possibly graft the bone to preserve and regenerate the support structure for the teeth. Antibiotics may be prescribed as well. These procedures are very predictable and are very successful in saving teeth for these patients. In extremely severe cases, the teeth may need to be extracted.

Susan opted for laser gum surgery due to the reduced downtime. The infected areas were accessed using a laser and were cleaned to remove the adherent plaque and bacteria, and bone was grafted—where possible—to provide help to regenerate the lost bone support for her teeth. Once we improved her gum pockets and the inflammation was gone, the orthodontist started straightening the tilted teeth and fixing the crowding in the front of Susan's mouth. While in braces, she was on a strict 3-month professional cleaning regimen with constant instructions and guidance to maintain excellent oral hygiene. The orthodontist helped upright the tilted molars and create room for dental implant replacement for her missing teeth.

We taught Susan how to properly maintain her teeth, and, as a healthy adult, she now has a full set of teeth that serve her well. In healthy patients, once the periodontitis is under control, regular periodontal checkups and good oral hygiene will keep the disease in check and prevent further damage to gums, bone, and teeth. Through managed treatment and maintenance, even advanced gum disease can be well-controlled. Studies have found that patients who get periodontal treatment and continue their regular professional cleanings lose fewer teeth. This is true for my patients. However, it is imperative for them to continue good oral hygiene and regular professional dental cleanings and dental care.

While the dental procedures to control periodontitis are the same for patients with and without an immune issue, periodontitis in patients with immune issues tends to reoccur because their bodies just cannot fight it. It is incredibly frustrating for these patients and for the periodontist or dentists who treat them.

Asha is one of these patients. When she came to see us, her gums were so enlarged that it was difficult for her to close her mouth. Her gums were red and bled easily, but while there was a little tenderness, Asha was still not really experiencing pain.

During our examination and review of medical history, we found out that Asha had recently had a kidney transplant and was taking cyclosporine, an immunosuppressant drug commonly used for kidney transplant patients. A side effect of Cyclosporine is that it causes gums to enlarge. If there is even a small amount of plaque present, the gums swell up and can grow incredibly large, sometimes covering the entire tooth.

Obviously, Asha's kidney disease was a bigger issue than her gum disease. In my practice, we work to find solutions that allow our patients to continue their medication regimens while we help them maintain their oral health. We consulted with her physician, and we performed gum surgery to trim her tissues to a normal level. Due to the amount of bleeding involved in this type of surgery, we used a laser to control the bleeding and performed the surgery in two visits, first on the gums in the upper jaw and then the lower jaw.

During her gum surgery, after the excess inflamed tissue was removed, we found a large amount of plaque and tartar. Because her gums were so large, it was impossible for Asha to properly clean her teeth. After the surgery, her gums were reduced to their normal healthy size, and we taught Asha how to brush and floss well and how to maintain good oral hygiene and dental health. We also set up a strict schedule of professional dental cleaning with our hygienist every two to three months.

She maintained this schedule for several years, and while some of the inflammation did come back, it was manageable. She was delighted to smile and eat again and not worry about bad breath and bleeding gums.

It is incredibly important for patients with periodontal disease to understand what is going on in the rest of their body and to be aware of any other sources of inflammation that need treatment. To control their periodontitis, they must also have all other medical conditions under control. It can be overwhelming for these patients to manage all their conditions simultaneously. That is why it is so important to have a team of medical and dental professionals working together with the patient to keep everything in balance.

For the majority of my patients struggling with multiple inflammatory diseases, I work with their physicians. However, with the increasing demands placed upon physicians these days, they are often hard to reach unless the situation is potentially life-threatening. Therefore, I now arm my patients with knowledge, encouraging them to take charge of their health and push their physicians to make sure that their blood sugar is under control, whether through nutrition, exercise, or medication.

I have many patients whose doctors have prescribed diet and exercise to control their diabetes instead of medications, but the patients are not following their doctors' advice. Because these patients visit my practice every three months for their periodontal checkups, they are seeing us more often than they see their physicians. They especially spend more time with the hygienists at my practice.

This gives us an opportunity to encourage these patients to recover their health through diet and exercise. We educate our patients on the importance of good overall health to help reduce inflammation. I have even started recommending some supplements for gut health and to encourage healthy weight.

Even though, as periodontists, we are trained to understand medical conditions that affect the rest of the body as well as the mouth, I am not a physician, so I do not treat medical conditions. I do advocate for the overall health of my patients and encourage them to learn how to manage their individual health needs. The information in this book comes from my experience with my patients in my practice and is intended for patients to understand the significance of gum health and how it can profoundly affect overall health. We can easily reduce inflammation in our body by simply seeing the dentist regularly for professional cleanings and dental care. This book attempts to present some of the latest trends in research that connect gum disease to major chronic illnesses, help patients have more productive conversations about holistic health, and build better partnerships with their dentists and physicians to solve specific patient health problems. This book should not be used to diagnose or treat any medical condition. For diagnosis or treatment of medical conditions, please consult your physician.

Gum disease is a chronic bacterial infection aggravated and perpetuated by inflammation. If left untreated, the inflammation continues until there is tooth loss. This inflammatory process can affect the rest of the body as well. Now that we have a basic understanding of the disease, we can dig deeper to learn how this insidious disease has profound effects on our overall health and longevity.

Chapter 2

UNDERSTANDING INFLAMMATION

In 2008, the American Academy of Periodontology brought together several leading experts to discuss inflammation and its role in the progression of disease. This gathering helped highlight the relationship between various diseases and suggested that inflammation might be the common denominator.

While chronic inflammation is not the only factor in gum disease and the other health conditions that this book addresses, it is the underlying problem that these conditions have in common.

What Is Inflammation?

Inflammation is the response of the immune system to bacterial infection or other offending agents in the body. During infections, white blood cells are recruited by the immune system to attack and kill the bacteria, and a natural result of that is inflammation. Therefore, inflammation is actually a sign that your immune system is doing its job. However, if the source of the problem remains untreated, inflammation can become a destructive force.

Inflammation can be acute or chronic:

Acute

Acute inflammation develops rapidly, usually within minutes, but it is generally short-lived. Think about a bee sting. The area around the sting swells quickly, but as long as you are not allergic to bees, the swelling normally subsides within a week. Many of the mechanisms that spring into action to destroy invading microbes switch gears to cart away dead cells and repair damaged ones. This cycle returns the affected area to a state of balance, and the inflammation dissipates.

Chronic

If the inflammation is caused by bacteria or another health condition that is left untreated, it may become chronic. When this happens, white blood cells, in an attempt to defeat the intrusive force, may produce chemicals that attack healthy tissues and organs. Blood vessels will become leaky, and then fluid will collect in the tissues causing swelling and bleeding.

A 2002 study by the National Institutes of Health (NIH) revealed that the chronic inflammatory process plays a central role in the most challenging diseases of our time, including rheumatoid arthritis, cancer, heart disease, diabetes, asthma, and even Alzheimer's. Today, it is believed that almost all disease, including cancer, is a result of underlying inflammation.

Gum disease is also a chronic inflammatory disease, and several studies have pointed to a connection between gum disease and other health issues in the body. The bacteria and plaque that cause gum disease create an inflammatory response in the mouth. This can cause an inflammatory reaction in other parts of the body. For example, if a person has heart disease or diabetes, untreated gum disease can make those conditions harder to control. The opposite may be true as well. If a diabetes patient has a lot of inflammation, it can make their periodontal disease worse due to the inflammatory response. Therefore, even if the causes are different, the chain reaction that inflammation sets off in the body has the same effect.

Common Causes of Chronic Inflammation

Acute inflammation is easy to spot. The inflamed area will be red and swollen, and the inflammation may cause fever and pain. However, *chronic* inflammation does not usually reveal itself as easily. It is a silent, destructive force, and you will not know that you have a chronic inflammatory condition unless you see a doctor. Medical tests, such as measuring C reactive protein (CRP), are often used to detect chronic inflammation.

Even though chronic inflammation is not easily detectable, any of these common causes may increase your risk of developing chronic inflammation and may indicate its presence:

- **Digestive problems:** Alcohol and certain medications can cause inflammation of the stomach, or gastritis.
- **Emotional stress:** Chronic emotional stress can cause the release of cortisol, a stress hormone, which plays an important role in causing inflammation in the body.
- **Physical stress:** Chronic physical stress, such as lack of sleep for several days or running a marathon, can also cause the release of cortisol that can increase inflammation.
- **Insulin resistance:** This condition is commonly linked to type 2 diabetes. The body's blood cells will have a reduced or missing response to insulin, resulting in a high blood glucose level. This may result in chronic low-grade inflammation in the body.
- **Chronic infection:** Chronic infections can also result in persistent Inflammation in the body.

- **Hormonal imbalance:** An imbalance of hormones, such as estrogen, progesterone, etc., can cause the production of cortisol, resulting in chronic inflammation. Hormonal imbalances can lead to chronic inflammation in pregnant or menopausal women.
- **Synthetic fibers and chemicals:** Synthetic materials such as latex can cause inflammation in people with sensitivities to these materials. Certain chemicals and allergens, if inhaled or touched, can also cause inflammation.
- **Poor diet:** Studies have shown that food materials such as sugar, processed meat, white flour, etc., can cause inflammation in the body, while foods such as fruits, vegetables, nuts, fish, and olive oil are usually associated with reduced inflammation. A study led by Anne Minihane found a relationship between gut health and inflammation and how early life nutrition can influence inflammation.
- **Food allergies:** Allergies to foods such as nuts, fish, etc., can cause inflammation in the body as well. Also, conditions such as celiac disease and an immune response to gluten result in chronic inflammation. In extreme cases, even a small exposure to allergens can cause an immediate inflammatory response that is life-threatening.

Sometimes a change in your health condition can trigger inflammation. The day that Linda came to my practice, she had generalized gum inflammation and bleeding. The inflammation had created a huge lump in her gums, and she was concerned that she might have cancer.

Linda was pregnant and nearing the end of her second trimester. According to a 2006 study of periodontal disease and pregnancy led by Yiorgos A. Bobetsis, it is not uncommon for pregnant women to experience gum inflammation due to hormonal imbalance. Increasing hormone levels can sometimes cause a localized gum growth. This is known as a pregnancy tumor, although it is not really a tumor. It is a gum enlargement commonly found in an area where there is excess plaque or tartar. It is usually in a plaque retention area that is difficult to brush or floss. These areas bleed easily and sometimes get ulcerated and tender.

We were able to remove the lump during Linda's visit, and as is standard practice, we sent the tissue to a lab to confirm that it was not cancerous. Since Linda was healthy—with no gum disease—we cleaned her teeth, and she returned to her regular dentist for checkups. After she had her baby, her gums returned to normal, and she had no more issues.

If you are experiencing any of the causes of inflammation listed above and visit your doctor, they may not initially discuss your symptoms in terms of inflammation. However, if a doctor tells you that you have high LDL, says you need to reduce your sugar intake, or begins asking if you are experiencing any of the other causes of inflammation listed above, ask questions and make sure the doctor fully explains any conditions they suspect you have that may increase inflammation. You should also ask your doctor about the steps you should take to maintain your health.

Reducing, Eliminating, or Preventing Inflammation

While some causes of chronic inflammation may be genetic, there are actions you can take to minimize your chances of developing chronic inflammation. Take care of yourself by engaging in the following healthy habits:

- Eat a healthy diet and get regular exercise to control obesity, blood sugar, and bad cholesterol (LDL).
- Eat foods high in antioxidants, and avoid or reduce foods, such as sugar, that cause inflammation.
- Visit your doctor and get regular tests for blood sugar, cholesterol, etc.
- Get regular dental checkups and professional cleanings. Brush your teeth a minimum of twice a day and floss daily to reduce gum inflammation.
- Use stress-reduction techniques such as meditation.

- Quit smoking to prevent gum disease and eliminate inflammation caused by nicotine.

If you are already managing one or more health conditions, making the changes above can seem daunting. The important thing is to pick one thing and start. Also, build your team. Engage your medical and dental team, other experts, and friends and family to help you implement healthy changes into your life. Remember that wherever you are on the health spectrum, you can make incremental changes that will improve your health and quality of life.

> *During my dental residency at The University of Texas in Houston, I met a patient with a true desire to live a healthier lifestyle. Don had been a heavy smoker for many years. By the time I met him, he had lost some of his teeth and had abscesses and bone loss.*
>
> *Smoking has a devastating impact on gum health. A significant number of my periodontitis patients are people dealing with the dental impacts of long-term smoking. I have dedicated an entire chapter on the harmful effects of smoking on the teeth and gums.*
>
> *We stressed the need to quit smoking for the success of treatment and to prevent the disease from coming back. Due to the extent of the damage, Don had to make a commitment to his health as well as a financial commitment. Even though he had limited means, Don traveled to Houston for several appointments at*

the dental school where I was completing my residency, and he also worked with his insurance company to help pay the cost.

All this effort motivated Don to quit smoking. He said to me, "I'm going to quit," and he did. We performed gum surgery on Don to save most of his teeth that were salvageable and extracted teeth that were beyond saving. We also performed extensive bone grafting to grow back the lost bone and placed dental implants to restore Don's missing teeth. All his first molars had to be replaced with dental implants. His smile improved, and he felt so much better after he quit smoking and we got his periodontitis under control. The inflammation disappeared, and he felt better overall.

Twenty years later, he showed up at my practice. He had broken a tooth and needed it repaired. After all that time, it was wonderful to see that he still was not smoking, and he had been getting regular cleanings and maintaining his teeth. The work we did was still intact. It was gratifying to know that the investment he made in improving his health had a sustaining impact on his life.

Understanding How Gum Disease and Other Health Conditions Intersect

Now that we have a basic understanding of gum disease and inflammation, the following chapters will attempt to explain how gum disease and inflammation impact these other chronic inflammatory conditions. While there are several diseases and conditions involved, we will mainly focus on the following:

- Adult-onset diabetes
- Cardiovascular disease and stroke
- Smoking, COPD, pneumonia, and sleep apnea
- Pregnancy and hormonal factors, preterm low-birth-weight babies, gestational diabetes
- Gut issues, obesity, metabolic disorders
- Alzheimer's, autism spectrum

The final chapter of the book will provide practical advice to help you manage your dental health.

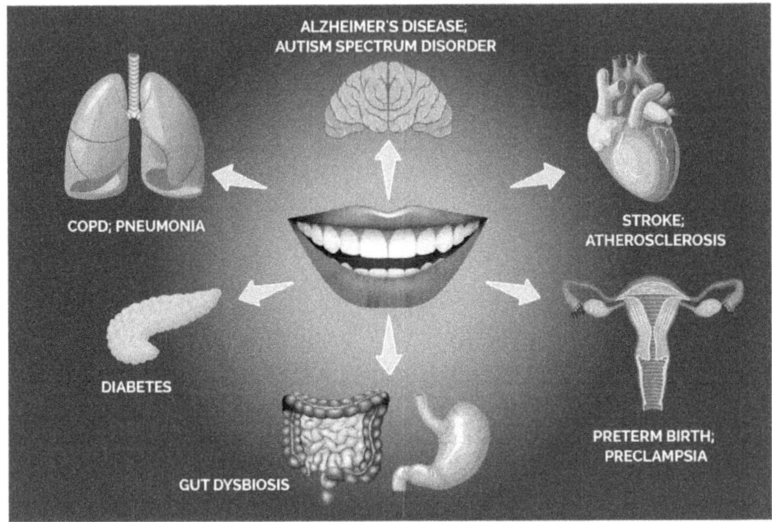

Diagrammatic representation of how gum disease may affect the rest of the body.

Chapter 3

ADULT-ONSET DIABETES

Adult-onset diabetes is the most prevalent chronic disease worldwide. According to a 2018 study by the American Diabetes Association, 10 percent of the global population suffers from the disease, with almost 29 million people diagnosed in the United States alone.

What Is Diabetes?

In a healthy body, carbohydrates are broken down into sugar, called glucose, which is released into the bloodstream. Insulin is a natural hormone that detects the sugar and helps the body either immediately use the sugar or store it for later use. In diabetes, the blood glucose level is too high due to a problem with insulin. This high blood sugar levels cause several health issues in the patient.

There are 2 main types of diabetes:

Type I: Patients with type 1 diabetes cannot produce insulin. The disease is more severe and requires patients to seek specialized medical treatments to manage their conditions.

Type II or Adult-onset diabetes: In these patients, their bodies are not capable of responding properly to insulin. Therefore, the sugar builds up in their bloodstream, and insulin production slows down.

The impact of Type I diabetes is beyond the scope of this book, and this book primarily focuses on adult-onset diabetes.

In 2005, the American Diabetes Association set the following three criteria for diagnosing diabetes with considerations for whether or not the person was fasting or had eaten two hours before testing:

- **Fasting** - Diabetes is present if a person's fasting blood sugar level is 126 or above, with a normal blood sugar level being less than 100.
- **Non-fasting (random testing)** - Diabetes is present if a person's non-fasting blood sugar level is greater than 200.
- **Food consumed two hours before testing** - Diabetes is present if the person's blood sugar level is greater than 200, with normal being less than 140.

High blood sugar levels can lead to issues with the eyes, nerves, kidneys, and heart, as well as the teeth and gums. Symptoms affecting teeth and gums in patients with uncontrolled diabetes include:

- **Less saliva and dry mouth** - Saliva washes away the bacteria and sticky food that can cause cavities and gum disease. It also carries antibodies that help protect the teeth and gums. Without the protection that saliva provides, there is an increased risk of cavities.
- **Swollen red gums and abscesses** - Gum disease is more prevalent in diabetics. Some studies suggest that gum disease may also raise blood sugar levels in both diabetics and non-diabetics.
- **Problems tasting food**
- **Delayed wound healing**
- **Increased infections in the mouth, like abscesses and cold sores**
- **Burning mouth syndrome**

How Gum Disease Affects Diabetes

Research performed by the American Dental Association in 2019 found that gum disease can affect diabetes in many ways. The study compared people with healthy gums to those with gum disease. People with gum disease have:

- Higher long-term blood sugar levels

- Higher risk of developing type II diabetes
- Higher risk of developing pregnancy (gestational) diabetes
- More difficulty controlling adult-onset diabetes
- Diabetics with gum disease may have a higher risk of:
  - Harm to the eyes
  - Damage to kidneys
  - Heart attack and stroke

Studies have also shown that severe gum disease is a strong predictor of mortality from ischemic heart disease and diabetic nephropathy (kidney disease due to diabetes) in people with adult-onset diabetes. A 2005 study found that periodontitis has an additional impact on these diseases in addition to the traditional risk factors.

How Diabetes Affects Gum Disease

The fact that patients with diabetes have more gum disease is well-established. These patients also experience more tooth loss. History of smoking, older age, infrequent visits to the dentist, brushing teeth less than once a day, a longer duration of diabetes, and complications due to diabetic neuropathy (nerve damage caused by diabetes) are all factors commonly associated with increased gum disease in diabetics.

A three-year study conducted by the National Health and Nutrition Examination Survey (NHANES) from 2009-2012 found that one-third of the diabetics studied had a severe form of gum disease and that adults aged 45 years or older, with poorly controlled diabetes, were three times more likely to have severe gum disease than those without diabetes.

Research has proven that bacteria in the mouths of diabetics are the same type of bacteria present in the mouths of non-diabetics. However, even though the bacteria are the same, the response of diabetic patients to the bacteria is very different. According to the American Academy of Periodontology, the function of immune cells is altered in diabetics. The white blood cells that gather to fight the toxins in the bacteria tend to over-respond and cause increased production of collagenase, enzymes, and toxins resulting in inflammation. Bacteria present in the mouth of a diabetic produce significantly more toxins than in non-diabetics; therefore, if left untreated, the gums and bone break down more quickly, and deeper pockets form. This cycle of destruction may lead to tooth loss and make it harder for the patient to manage their diabetes.

How Gum Disease Affects Diabetic Control

There is some evidence suggesting that when a patient with gum disease does normal activities, like chewing and toothbrushing, toxins in the gums leak into the bloodstream. This causes a reaction from the body's defense system which produces chemicals that have harmful effects on the body, one of which is raising your blood sugar.

Several studies have shown that severe gum disease in non-insulin-dependent diabetics makes blood sugar control more difficult; therefore, severe gum disease is a significant risk factor for diabetics. Diabetics with untreated severe gum disease have six times the risk of their blood sugar control worsening over time as opposed to diabetics without severe gum disease.

Treatment and Prevention

I see the impact of adult-onset diabetes every day. It is very important for people struggling with this disease to learn how to control and manage it. It is equally important for them to know that, with help, they *can* manage it.

> *Kerry, a recently divorced, 60-year-old woman came to see me because she wanted to start dating again. She was dealing with bad breath and uncontrolled adult-onset diabetes and was trying to take care of herself. Her x-rays and exam showed severe bone loss, loose teeth, and swollen gums, with infected areas, abscesses, and deep gum pockets around some teeth. Kerry had no pain and was not aware of the level of destruction inside her mouth. She thought she just needed mouthwash. As we pointed to the damage on*

the x-rays, we explained that she had advanced gum disease, and, if it was not treated, she would soon need dentures. We also told her that, like diabetes, gum disease is a chronic, silent disease. Often, by the time it is found, a lot of damage has been done.

Kerry was motivated to take care of her gums and went through comprehensive periodontal treatment. The inflammation subsided, her gums were pink and healthy, the abscesses healed, and her bad breath disappeared. Kerry understood the seriousness of having both diabetes and gum disease. She focused on improving her diet and getting regular exercise. She also maintained proper dental care and made other lifestyle changes to improve her health. Her blood sugar stabilized, and she felt energetic and ready for the next phase of her life.

My focus in regard to diabetes is to understand how the disease impacts a patient's mouth and how treatment can influence diabetic control. The good news is that research shows that the treatment of gum disease helps improve glycemic control in diabetics and may help reduce HbA1c. HbA1c is a measurement that shows how level a patient's blood sugar has been for the two to three months prior. The American Diabetes Association says that if your HbA1c level is between 5.7 and 6.5, then you are considered pre-diabetic. But if it is 6.5 or higher, you are considered diabetic.

Testing your HbA1c level is different than the fasting blood test you get during your annual physical. A fasting blood test will show only the blood sugar level at that moment in time. So, if you do a crash course healthy diet a few days before your physical, you may get a passing grade from your doctor, but you also may not get the full picture of your health. During your physical, make sure to tell your doctor about any symptoms you may be experiencing, and if your fasting blood sugar is above 100, discuss whether or not an HbA1c blood test is warranted.

If a person with adult-onset diabetes has gum disease, as long as their blood sugar level is under control, their periodontal treatment can be conducted and maintained as effectively as a person without adult-onset diabetes. However, if their blood level gets out of control, some dental treatments will not be as effective until they regain control of their blood sugar.

Patients with severe adult-onset diabetes struggle with blood sugar control. Oral medication is usually ineffective, so they have to take insulin. Sometimes, even with this stronger medication, it may be difficult to manage the disease.

> *Severe gum disease in a person with severe adult-onset diabetes is also difficult to control. Jonathon came to my practice as a referral from his regular dentist who had recognized the telltale signs of severe gum disease. While recording his medical history, we*

discovered Jonathon had adult-onset diabetes and was taking insulin. Our first treatment to bring his gum disease under control was to perform a deep cleaning. At the same time, we consulted with his medical doctor and requested blood work results to help us decide if Jonathon was a candidate for surgery.

Most severe patients are treated in two steps. The first step is a non-surgical deep cleaning, and the second step is gum surgery. In patients with both severe adult-onset diabetes and severe gum disease, I have found that even though we can reduce the bacteria through deep cleanings, the surgery necessary to completely eradicate the infection is not always an option due to uncontrolled blood sugar levels. Therefore, before we plan gum surgery on any of these patients, we consult with their doctor to ensure that the patient's blood sugar is under control. This is a necessary step because performing surgery on a diabetic with uncontrolled blood sugar can lead to a further spread of infection that can cause fever and impact the healing process.

Jonathon's doctor told us that his blood sugar was very erratic. Therefore, our treatment plan was to maintain Jonathon's gum disease non-surgically. Unfortunately, this is a compromise situation because with severe gum disease, there is no way to completely remove the infection caused by the disease without surgery.

We performed the deep cleaning and encouraged Jonathon to eat a healthy diet, get regular exercise, take his medication, and practice good dental hygiene. We also performed periodontal cleanings on Jonathon every three months. This treatment plan was designed to allow Jonathon time to get his blood sugar under control so we could perform surgery and remove the infection.

The deep cleaning slowed the growth of the infection. But it is very difficult for severe diabetics to control their blood sugar levels, and Jonathon was not successful. Without the necessary surgery, the infection continued to grow, and, due to his diabetes, his immune system could not fight the infection well. This combination further deteriorated Jonathon's teeth and gums, even with maintenance. Within two years, we noticed that some of Jonathon's teeth were starting to loosen and needed to be extracted.

For patients with severe, uncontrolled diabetes, extra precautions must be taken. We consulted with Jonathon's doctor again to see if his insulin dosage could be increased or his medical treatment temporarily changed to control his blood sugar so we could perform the extractions. Sometimes this is possible, but Jonathon's doctor told us that the infection in Jonathon's body was preventing control of his blood sugar and recommended that we go ahead and remove the teeth. We gave Jonathon antibiotics and performed the extractions.

Over time, we ended up extracting all of Jonathon's teeth and fitting him for dentures. It took a long time for him to heal, but once all his teeth were extracted, the source of bacteria in his mouth was gone. Therefore, the gum disease was gone. He was not happy to lose his teeth but was grateful we helped him maintain his teeth for several years.

We could not perform implant surgery on Jonathon or give him fixed teeth. Patients with uncontrolled diabetes do not succeed with these treatments. Teeth are naturally surrounded and supported by tissue; implants are not. This makes implants very susceptible to infection. As long as the blood sugar level is controlled and dental hygiene is maintained, the plaque will be removed, and there will be no problems. However, for patients with uncontrolled diabetes, the plaque buildup causes the bacteria to aggressively invade the gums and attack the supporting bone. The immune system does not stop the onslaught because the cells in diabetics tend to be hyper-responsive and produce toxins that result in more bone loss. As the bone deteriorates, the implant will become loose and must be removed.

Another issue with implants in patients like Jonathon is that the gum disease has progressed to a point that there is not enough bone structure to support an implant. In patients with controlled diabetes, it is possible to do grafts and grow the bone back. However, in patients with severe, uncontrolled diabetes, the grafts become infected easily, and sometimes the bone loss is so pronounced that it is not possible to grow it all back. Therefore, patients with severe, uncontrolled diabetes are not good candidates for implants, and dentures are their best option. Jonathan has decided to control his blood sugar and return to our office to get dental implants and fixed teeth. We are excited to see him motivated and know this will help his overall health in the long run.

Whether or not you have diabetes, it is important to keep your teeth and gums healthy.

- Brush your teeth gently twice a day with a soft-bristle brush and toothpaste
- Clean in between your teeth with floss or an interdental brush
- See a dentist regularly for cleanings

If you have adult-onset diabetes, keeping your gums healthy may help you control your blood sugar levels. It may also help lower your risk of complications such as kidney disease and blindness due to diabetes. If you have been diagnosed with diabetes and gum disease, it is important to partner with medical and periodontal professionals to control and manage both. If you have lapsed in your periodontal maintenance, you may need periodontal treatment. Periodontal treatment usually involves deep cleaning the gum pockets to remove the bacteria from the root surfaces. Severe cases may require gum surgery to clean out the deep infection. Antibiotics may be prescribed as well. With treatment, the gum inflammation will subside, and combined with diabetes treatment and management, some patients have seen insulin sensitivity restored with improved metabolic control.

In 2006, Brian Mealey concluded that diabetes clearly increases the risk of gum disease. We also know that gum disease can affect blood sugar; however, we do not have a full understanding of the impacts and how they take place. Further research is in progress to clarify this aspect of the relationship between gum disease and diabetes. In the meantime, we do understand that there is a strong connection, and we also know that proper care of teeth and gums helps diabetics control their blood sugar. Therefore, endocrinologists and physicians recommend that diabetic patients take care of their gums to reduce overall inflammation and help manage their diabetes.

Chapter 4

CARDIOVASCULAR DISEASE AND STROKE

In the most basic terms, coronary heart disease—also known as cardiovascular disease—means that the arteries leading to the heart are incapable of delivering enough oxygen-rich blood. It is the result of partial or complete blockage of the blood flow caused by plaque buildup in the arteries. According to the NIH, heart disease is the leading cause of death throughout the world.

The medical term for plaque buildup is atherosclerosis. You may have also heard this referred to as "hardening of the arteries." The plaque is a combination of fats, cholesterol, and other substances that "harden" and stick to arterial walls. This can narrow or block the arteries, thus restricting blood flow. Systemic inflammation is increasingly being recognized as a risk factor for a number of diseases, including atherosclerosis. Research indicates that C-reactive protein

(CRP) plays a role in the development of atherosclerosis. CRP forms in the liver and is released into the bloodstream any time there is inflammation in the body.

One of the major risk factors for heart disease is high cholesterol levels that encourage plaque formation in arteries. The human body's response to bacteria in gum disease may also be related to atherosclerosis and coronary events. The bacteria can result in inflammation, and since CRP is released when severe inflammation is present in the body, studies suggest a correlation between severe gum disease and atherosclerosis.

Effects of Periodontal Disease on Heart Disease

Viral and bacterial infections may contribute to heart disease, according to recent studies. One study found that the odds of a patient with gum disease getting heart disease are as high as 5.74, or more than five times greater than the control group. Other studies associate severe gum disease with a higher risk for arterial plaque formation and warned that this could lead to a variety of coronary events including:

- Myocardial infarction - Heart damage caused by blocked blood vessels
- Ischemic stroke - Stroke caused by a lack of blood supply to the brain due to blockage in arteries

- Peripheral arterial disease - Blockage of any blood vessel which leads to another medical issue, such as gangrene, which is decaying tissue due to the loss of blood supply

While the exact nature of the connection between infection and heart disease is yet to be identified, there is significant evidence that the connection exists:

1. Higher levels of low-density lipoprotein (LDL), bad cholesterol, and lower levels of high-density lipoprotein (HDL), good cholesterol, in the bloodstream increase the likelihood of arterial blockage. Multiple studies have found that severe gum disease is associated with increased levels of LDL, total cholesterol, and triglycerides. Furthermore, these studies show that severe gum disease decreases the level and potency of HDL. Deeper pockets, which denote severe gum disease, were associated with both total cholesterol and LDL cholesterol levels.
2. Other studies suggest that severe gum disease increases the levels of circulating cytokines, or toxins, and inflammatory substances in the blood. This includes CRP, which appears to increase the risk of heart disease. These inflammatory substances can damage the lining of the blood vessels, causing platelets and other cells to stick to the damaged lining. Over time, cholesterol, cells, bacteria, and other

substances form into plaque, which may result in atherosclerosis or arterial blockage.

3. Mouth bacteria may encourage the production of antibodies that can damage and cause blockage in blood vessels. This may cause even more damage and plaque formation in arteries.

This mounting evidence is leading doctors to increasingly identify severe gum disease as a factor in the heart health of their patients.

Stroke

Strokes can occur in the brain when a blood clot prevents oxygen from getting to the brain or when a blood vessel in the brain bursts. Anyone can have a stroke at any age, but the risk for stroke increases due to age, sex, and ethnicity. Some risks are attributed to poor lifestyle choices, including smoking, excessive alcohol consumption, and a lack of exercise. Other health conditions like heart disease, high blood pressure, high cholesterol, or diabetes are risk factors for stroke. A major contributing factor for stroke is the narrowing of arteries caused by atherosclerosis. As we discussed earlier in the chapter, studies show that severe gum disease may be a contributing factor to atherosclerosis, and therefore, it may also be a contributing factor for stroke.

Stroke and gum disease have a lot in common, most significantly, inflammation. With so many Americans affected by both conditions, it is important to recognize that the two may have connections. By knowing the facts, you and your medical and dental professionals can make better decisions about how to reduce your risk of developing these life-threatening diseases.

For patients struggling with both cardiovascular disease and severe gum disease, it is never too soon to act. Atherosclerosis is a ticking time bomb, and the best treatment is prevention.

> *William was referred to me by his cardiologist. William was a high-risk heart patient with an elevated risk of stroke and severe gum disease. His CRP levels indicated that he had a dangerous level of inflammation, and his cardiologist was initiating an aggressive treatment plan that included eliminating the inflammation caused by his severe gum disease.*
>
> *The treatment for William's gum disease was planned in two phases. During his first visit, we performed a deep cleaning to control the infection and inflammation in his gums. William understood the seriousness of his gum disease and was very cooperative with the treatment. We set his next appointment for four weeks later to do a follow-up exam and determine if he was a candidate for surgery. However, William did not show up for his next appointment. When we called to check on him, we found that he had suffered a stroke and passed away.*

> *I felt sadness for William and his family. There may have been an opportunity to treat his severe gum disease, reduce inflammation, and possibly reduce his chances of getting a stroke. As doctors, we do all we can to help our patients at whatever stage they are when we meet them, but for patients like William, we always wish we had met them earlier.*

We know that inflammation leads to atherosclerosis. Atherosclerosis makes it more difficult for blood to flow to and from the heart, which can lead to stroke. In patients with severe gum disease, bacteria that enter through the gums may spread to the blood vessels and contribute to plaque buildup which thickens, or narrows, blood vessels as the plaque increases. We know this because the same bacteria present in gum disease has been found in arterial plaque. Arterial plaque decreases cardiovascular health and increases the risk of stroke. Pieces of arterial plaque can break off the arterial walls, travel through the blood vessels, and become lodged, blocking off the blood to areas of the body. Any tissue that does not receive the blood will immediately start to decay. Therefore, blockage of a blood vessel in any area of the body will result in a major medical event. If the plaque becomes lodged in a carotid artery, the arteries that supply oxygen-rich blood to the brain, a stroke will occur.

Several studies have shown that gum disease is associated with increased markers of inflammation, which are themselves indicators of stroke risk. It has also been found that bacteria from infected pockets in the gums can enter the bloodstream during activities such as chewing or tooth brushing. Mouth bacteria were first identified in plaque in the carotid arteries, which supply blood to the brain and head.

A 2018 study led by Dr. Sen Souvik confirmed a connection between severe gum disease and incident stroke risk, particularly cardioembolic and thrombotic stroke. A cardioembolic stroke occurs when the heart pumps unwanted materials into the blood-brain circulation, resulting in the blockage of a blood vessel in the brain and damage to the brain tissue. A thrombotic stroke is a type of ischemic stroke that occurs when a blood clot, also called a thrombus, blocks blood flow through the artery in which it formed. The blood clot may block the flow of oxygen-rich blood to a portion of the brain, resulting in long-term brain damage. The study concluded that regular dental care to prevent gum disease may lower the risk for stroke from plaque, with mouth bacteria as a contributing factor.

> *By the time Martin came to see us, he had been struggling with heart disease for many years. He had suffered a previous stroke and was taking blood thinners. His dentist had referred him to us for treatment of his gum disease. Since Martin was taking blood thinners, we set his treatment as non-surgical until we could consult with his doctor.*

If a patient has heart disease and has suffered a recent stroke, no surgical treatments can be performed for at least six months to a year after the event until the patient is fully recovered. Martin's stroke had been two years prior and he was cleared for periodontal surgery by his physician. Based on his initial appointment, we felt he was a candidate for surgery. The second hurdle was the blood thinners which may cause increased bleeding and bruising. It is possible to perform periodontal surgery on a patient taking blood thinners, but we have to proceed very carefully, working on only a few areas at a time, and making sure that we can control any bleeding. We warn the patient that they may get a bruise, and after the surgery, we monitor them closely.

The other option for patients on blood thinners is to stop the medication before the surgery. This is risky for some patients because the patient needs the blood thinners to prevent blood clots from forming. However, Martin was responding well to the treatment for his heart disease, and his doctor gave the clearance to stop the blood thinners five days before the surgery.

Even with the blood thinners stopped, we were mindful of Martin's condition and performed conservative and minimally invasive surgery. Fortunately, this was enough, and we successfully cleaned out all the infection. Martin resumed taking his blood thinner medication the day after the surgery.

Martin is doing very well with both his heart disease and gum disease maintenance. He has regular periodontal maintenance cleanings, observes a good dental hygiene regimen, and works closely with us and his cardiologist to keep both his heart disease and gum disease in check. I am happy to report that there are many success stories like Martin's.

There are factors associated with a higher risk of stroke that are not preventable. Some of these factors include type 1 diabetes, narrow blood vessels, high levels of bad cholesterol, etc. However, gum disease is preventable and is treatable.

Treatment and Prevention

Understanding the connection between inflammation and chronic disease and reducing the inflammation caused by disease has become a major focus in both the dental and medical professions. As a growing number of studies find links between severe gum disease and high-risk factors for cardiovascular disease, dental healthcare professionals are increasingly being recognized for the important role they play in protecting their patients' overall wellness.

Treatment of gum disease with routine scaling and root planing to remove the plaque and sometimes giving antibiotics to kill the bacteria has been found to reduce inflammatory markers such as CRP. In severe cases with no other options, the extraction of all teeth has resulted in a significant reduction in CRP levels. This is further evidence that severe gum disease is a contributing factor in these inflammatory markers.

> *Gina was an elderly woman who came to our office with her adult daughter. Gina had bleeding gums, loose teeth, and abscesses. She was experiencing a lot of pain. Her daughter was worried and explained that she wanted her mom to be able to eat again.*
>
> *Gina's condition was further complicated by a history of heart disease and uncontrolled diabetes. She had previously suffered a heart attack and was taking several medications, including blood thinners. She was considered at risk for another heart attack due to the high levels of inflammatory markers—including CRP—in her blood.*
>
> *We consulted with Gina's physicians, and due to the severity of her multiple conditions, we decided that the best course of treatment was to extract all of her teeth and give her dentures. Removing the painful, infected teeth gave Gina a new lease on life. The smile that had long abandoned her returned, and she started eating healthier and taking better care of herself. We were so pleased the day that her daughter told us*

that Gina's blood tests showed lower CRP levels and a lower risk of heart attack.

There is a large body of evidence to indicate that CRP levels are elevated in patients with severe gum disease, but further investigation is required to support periodontal treatment as a means of controlling systemic inflammation in the general population. However, with more and more studies linking inflammation to a variety of chronic diseases, there is a growing acceptance among both dental and medical professionals, including the American Heart Association (AHA), that there is a strong connection between severe gum disease and heart disease.

The AHA has published guidelines for the treatment of gum disease for patients with known heart conditions. This includes using antibiotics before treatment in some patients in coordination with the patient's doctor.

Patients who are susceptible to heart disease, stroke, or gum disease already have all the risk factors that complicate treatment. If only one condition is treated, the other conditions will prevent the management of the inflammation present, and the treatment will fail. This is why it is vital to control all the conditions that are contributing to the inflammation. Severe gum disease is one of these conditions because we know that the toxins formed in the gums can enter the bloodstream and travel to other parts of the body as contributing factors in the buildup of arterial plaque.

If you have cardiovascular risk factors, like high blood pressure or obesity, work with your physician and take steps to eliminate these issues. Make sure to also maintain proper oral hygiene with regular dental cleanings to prevent gum disease. If you have been diagnosed with both severe gum disease and heart disease, you should work closely with both your doctor and periodontist to monitor your condition because you are at an increased risk for a medical event. Make sure that your doctor knows about your severe gum disease and that your periodontist knows about your heart disease and any other health conditions you may have. Talk to them both about how you can reduce the inflammation in your body caused by your health conditions. By taking these steps, you are building a team of professionals that will help you receive the specific care you need.

Improving your diet by reducing salt, red meat, and foods high in saturated fat and cholesterol is another step you can take to help fight inflammation and atherosclerosis. Remember that many processed foods are high in salt, saturated fat, and cholesterol, so be sure to read the labels. Eat more natural foods, including fruits and vegetables, nuts and seeds, and olive oil or nut oils in place of butter. Probiotics and prebiotics have also been shown to help with reducing cardiovascular disease by reducing inflammation.

Exercise is another important part of your overall wellness. However, before starting any exercise program, work with your doctor to determine a plan that is right for you.

Research in modern dentistry is leading to advances both in the comfort and overall wellness of patients. For many years, traditional surgery with a scalpel and sutures was the only option for treating severe gum disease. The treatment was painful and required a long recovery period. Fortunately, in 2016, a laser treatment option was approved by the Food and Drug Administration (FDA). Laser surgery may be a less painful and more successful treatment with shorter recovery periods.

Even with the many studies that have provided clues to the connection between gum disease and cardiovascular disease, additional large-scale studies are needed to fully understand this link. However, based on what we know today, healthcare providers are beginning to include gum disease as a factor in the treatment of their heart patients.

Chapter 5

RESPIRATORY CONDITIONS

Smoking and Chronic Obstructive Lung Disease (COPD), Sleep Apnea

According to the CDC, cigarette smoking is the leading preventable cause of death in the United States. More than 48,000 Americans die each year from smoking-related illnesses. While the human respiratory system is an amazing cleaning factory that filters irritants and allows the body to absorb oxygen while expelling carbon dioxide, it is not designed to manage the regular ingestion of the smoke and chemicals in tobacco products.

When we breathe in air, it flows into the bronchi, or air tubes, and down into the lungs. In the lungs, the bronchi branch off into smaller tubes called bronchioles. At the tip of the bronchioles are the alveoli, or air sacs. The alveoli filter the air, releasing the oxygen into the bloodstream while pushing the carbon dioxide back into the lungs to release when we breathe out.

When smoke goes into the lungs, the tar in the smoke begins damaging the alveoli, and over time, some of the alveoli will stop functioning. This diminishes the capacity of the lungs to take in air, release oxygen into the bloodstream, and expel carbon dioxide. Therefore, the body is deprived of oxygen and also has a higher level of carbon dioxide.

While smoking may be viewed by many as an addictive habit, it is, in fact, a disease that is the leading risk factor in the development of multiple chronic diseases, including chronic obstructive lung disease (COPD). According to the CDC and the American Lung Association, COPD is the combination of two chronic diseases, bronchitis and emphysema, and may at times include asthma. Chronic bronchitis is severe inflammation that narrows or blocks the bronchi, or air tubes, that lead into the lungs. Patients with chronic bronchitis have difficulty breathing and may need to frequently use an inhaler to open up the bronchi. Emphysema is damage to the alveoli. When the alveoli are damaged, the lungs cannot work to capacity, and the patient struggles with constant shortness of breath. COPD is characterized by the chronic blockage of airflow and breathing-related problems.

While air pollution, second-hand smoke, a history of childhood respiratory infections, genetic factors, and heredity are among other risk factors for COPD, the CDC reports that cigarette smoking is a contributing factor in nearly 80 percent of COPD cases.

Smoking is so impactful that the American Surgical Association (ASA) includes it as a significant health condition in classifying patients. The **ASA score** is a subjective assessment of a patient›s overall health based on the following five classes:

ASA I - A normal healthy patient who is a non-smoker, with minimal or no alcohol use

ASA II - A patient with a mild disease impacting the body but one which does not limit function

- Examples include, but are not limited to, current smoker, moderate alcohol drinker, pregnant, obese (BMI over 30 for more than 60 weeks), and a history of cardiovascular disease (present for more than 3 months)

ASA III - A patient with one or more moderate-to-severe systemic diseases causing functional limitations

- Examples include, but are not limited to, uncontrolled diabetes, high blood pressure, COPD, morbid obesity (a BMI of 40 or more), active hepatitis, alcohol dependence or abuse, an implanted pacemaker, etc.

ASA IV - A patient with severe systemic disease that is a constant threat to life

- Examples include, but are not limited to, uncontrolled COPD, heart failure, etc.

ASA V - A critically ill patient who is not expected to survive without an operation

- Examples include, but are not limited to, heart surgery, brain surgery, blood clot in the brain or lungs, etc.

COPD is one of the leading causes of death in the United States. In 2020, healthypeople.gov reported that 14.8 million Americans had been diagnosed with COPD. A particular danger to COPD patients is developing pneumonia. Pneumonia often begins with a small cough with little to no fever but may quickly lead to hospitalization for a COPD patient.

Research has concluded that tooth decay, mouth bacteria, and poor oral hygiene are risk factors for COPD-related pneumonia and that improving oral health may help reduce the occurrence of pneumonia.

> *Lou was a 58-year-old patient referred to our office by his physician. He was a heavy smoker, suffered from COPD, and had experienced several episodes of pneumonia. The physician wanted us to evaluate Lou for*

gum disease and treat it, as needed, in hopes that it would relieve some of his COPD symptoms.

Lou had severe gum disease with deep pockets, bone loss, loose teeth, and bleeding gums. We recommended starting with non-surgical periodontal treatment, which included deep scaling and root planing, antibiotics, and meticulous oral hygiene instructions. We explained to Lou that this initial phase of treatment was intended to reduce the bacteria and inflammation to prepare his mouth for the next phase, the surgical treatment. We also recommended a program to help him stop smoking.

Lou finished the non-surgical treatment but failed to follow up after that. We attempted several times to reach him to complete the treatment. Two years later, we received a letter from his physician telling us that Lou had, unfortunately, passed away from complications of pneumonia.

It is often very difficult for patients with multiple medical issues to manage all that is going wrong. It can be overwhelming. This is why it is so necessary to surround yourself with medical and dental professionals who can help implement a step-by-step program designed specifically for your needs.

Smoking and Gum Disease

Numerous studies over the past 20 years have shown that smoking is a major risk factor in the development of gum disease and may be responsible for more than half of gum disease cases among adults in the United States.

Smoking makes gum disease worse by changing the bacteria, allowing aggressive bacteria to grow, and influencing the immune response to the bacteria. Recent reports have documented a higher prevalence of certain microorganisms in smokers. Smokers showed greater numbers of bad bacteria, especially in pockets. Smoking also affects the cells that cause immune response and inflammation.

> *Jen had been smoking a pack of cigarettes a day for 20 years when she came to our office with a toothache. During our examination, we found severe gum disease with loose teeth and red, swollen gums. Our recommended treatment plan included gum surgery to save her teeth and extracting some teeth that were beyond saving.*
>
> *Jen was very upset about the extractions because she was barely 40 years old. I sat down and explained the damage to her gums and teeth caused by smoking. She wanted to make sure she would not lose any more teeth, so, with medication and support from her doctor, Jen started a program to quit smoking.*

It was very difficult for Jen to quit, but eventually, she succeeded. We cleaned out the infection, grafted, and grew new bone and helped save her teeth. We then gave Jen implants to replace the extracted teeth. She regained her health, her smile, and her confidence. Jen has been seeing our hygienist for cleanings every three months, religiously, and has been successfully maintaining good health and has not lost a single tooth since then. Losing some of her teeth was a wake-up call that encouraged her to make a change and lead a happier, healthier life.

COPD and Gum Disease

Studies on dental health and COPD have examined factors such as bone loss around the teeth, plaque and tartar build-up, and other evidence of severe gum disease. Other studies have examined the impacts of cigarette smoking and dental health on COPD.

COPD can be exacerbated with any infection. Therefore, effective management of COPD involves the prevention and reduction of infections, including infections in the mouth related to gum disease. The mouth of a COPD patient with uncontrolled gum disease is teeming with bacteria that can be aspirated into the lower respiratory tract, increasing the risk of respiratory infection and death.

Research suggests four possible reasons for the presence of oral bacteria in connection to respiratory problems:

1. Bacteria that cause lung infections could grow in dental plaque and cause lung disease.
2. Gum disease-associated enzymes may destroy protective salivary coatings on the tissues, which will allow an increased number of bacteria to stick to the bronchi and cause disease. Infection may spread from the back of the mouth directly into the throat, or infection may spread from the bacteria entering the blood vessels and traveling to the lungs.
3. In patients with untreated gum disease, a large variety of toxins produced by the inflammatory cells can occur. When the patient swallows, these toxins and molecules may cause problems in the airway and the lungs.
4. The aspiration of mouth secretions, food, or stomach contents, or breathing in bacteria as an aerosol may increase infections in the bronchi and lungs.

While more research on the connection between gum disease and COPD is needed, we know that aspirating mouth secretions is the most common way that bad bacteria associated with gum disease enter the bronchi and lungs, causing infection and escalating respiratory issues. There is also evidence that connects tooth loss due to gum disease with a higher risk of a person developing COPD.

Tooth Loss and COPD

Tooth loss significantly changes the association between cigarette smoking and COPD. Understanding the connection between cigarette smoking, oral health, and COPD—particularly as they relate to tooth loss, infection, and inflammation—is essential for COPD patients.

Current smokers with all their teeth removed are almost seven times more likely to report COPD than people who do not smoke and have not lost their teeth. Remarkably, people with one to five teeth removed are significantly more likely to have COPD than people who have never smoked and do not have any tooth loss. These findings suggest that the association between cigarette smoking and COPD becomes stronger with increased tooth loss. Therefore, greater attention may be needed to promote the importance of good oral health in maintaining healthy lungs and bodies, including education about proper oral hygiene, the dangers of smoking, and encouraging access to preventive and therapeutic dental care.

Severe gum disease is a leading cause of local and inflammatory effects throughout the body, including increased levels of C-reactive protein (CRP) and toxins in the bloodstream. In the presence of widespread, uncontrolled gum disease, the toxins in cigarettes, such as nicotine, and the toxins produced by a strong immune response result in increased inflammation, gum damage, and tooth loss.

If the food and bacteria are aspirated into the lungs, it can cause further damage and infection.

Treatment and Recommendations

A large proportion of adult gum disease and COPD may be avoided through the prevention and cessation of cigarette smoking. After decades of smoking, quitting may seem impossible. However, success is achievable with the right program and the right support.

The Role of the Patient

1. Quit smoking
2. Seek treatment of periodontal disease
3. Get regular dental cleanings to prevent a recurrence
4. Practice good dental hygiene
5. Visit your doctor and follow medical advice for managing COPD symptoms

The Role of Dental and Health Professionals

1. Identify tobacco users
2. Advise the patient to quit smoking
3. Assess and evaluate the patient's readiness to quit smoking
4. Offer assistance to help the patient quit smoking
5. Follow up on the patient's efforts to quit smoking

Behavioral therapy that includes lifestyle changes, counseling, and medications, as well as low dose nicotine, like the patch, has been shown to increase the success rate for quitting smoking. Using the patch with counseling has proven twice as successful as counseling alone. A program of prescribed medication while also using the patch can be very helpful for heavy smokers or smokers who have tried many times but failed to quit smoking.

Periodontal Treatment in Smokers

Periodontal treatment and periodontal surgery help remove bacteria, reduce inflammation, and save teeth in all patients including smokers. But studies have shown periodontal treatment may be less effective for smokers than non-smokers. Because smokers take longer to heal after periodontal treatment, antibiotics are often recommended to improve the treatment results. Many patients who smoke have successful outcomes with periodontal treatment but have a higher chance of disease recurrence if they continue smoking heavily.

In addition to the obvious health benefits of not smoking, studies show that former smokers heal and respond to treatment as well as non-smokers. Former smokers may even be able to achieve the same success with implants as patients who never smoked.

For patients with severe gum disease and COPD, periodontal treatment may reduce mouth bacteria, therefore reducing the frequency of COPD complications. As a result of regular dental cleanings and good oral hygiene practices in COPD patients help prevent bacteria from entering the lungs and causing infection. Controlling gum disease and saving teeth will also help in better chewing efficiency and is extremely important to prevent any aspiration. Also, replacing the missing teeth with a fixed solution like dental implants may help prevent these problems.

While more studies are needed to help us fully understand the connection between gum disease and COPD, we know that a connection exists. Patients at high risk of developing COPD can lower their risk by practicing good dental hygiene, having regular professional dental cleanings, quitting smoking, and moving forward with a healthier lifestyle. Patients who have been diagnosed with both gum disease and COPD should work closely with their dental and healthcare professionals to prevent infection through regular dental and medical treatment and maintenance.

Obstructive Sleep Apnea

Any airway discussion would not be complete without discussing obstructive sleep apnea (OSA). Sleep apnea is a potentially serious sleep disorder in which breathing repeatedly stops and starts. Sleep apnea is more commonly seen in males, with prevalence ranging from 5-28%. If you snore loudly and feel tired even after a full night's sleep, you might have sleep apnea. It has been associated with an increased risk for development of disorders, such as coronary heart disease, hypertension, stroke, congestive cardiac failure, and atherosclerosis, as well as impaired glucose tolerance and insulin resistance. Although the exact mechanism of how sleep apnea leads to complications is uncertain, it has been suggested that reduced oxygen caused by sleep apnea may cause inflammation. Treatment today is mostly focused on relieving the obstruction. There are non-surgical and surgical treatment options for OSA. Some patients with sleep apnea may benefit by using oral appliances to move the mandible forward (mandibular advancement devices) and CPAP therapy. Others may require surgery to remove excessive oral tissue that blocks airways during sleep.

Risk factors for periodontitis, such as sex, age, smoking, obesity, and diabetes are also relatively common in patients with obstructive sleep apnea. It has been shown in some studies that patients with sleep apnea had four times more gum disease than the national average. This increased periodontal disease may be related to mouth breathing that results in drying and irritation of the gums. Also lack of sleep affects the well-being of the patient and reduces the immune response causing increased susceptibility to gum disease.

Since the bacteria in gum disease are capable of causing inflammation and worsening any underlying inflammatory conditions, it can potentially worsen sleep apnea. Obstructive sleep apnea and periodontal disease could be associated due to the fact that both diseases share the same risk factors. Also, both conditions are caused by inflammatory response.

> *Carl was referred to us with severe gum disease. He was overweight and had high blood pressure. On examination, he had severe bone loss and deep gum pockets on all his teeth. His teeth were severely worn down, and he had several loose teeth. He had a large tongue and flared front teeth. He was interested in treating his gum disease and eventually getting braces. On questioning, he reported not sleeping well, and his wife mentioned loud snoring. We suspected sleep apnea and explained the need for a referral and a sleep study. We worked on treating his gum disease with surgery and helped control his infection and inflammation. We placed him on a 3-month professional maintenance cleaning at our office. He saw an ENT who specialized in the treatment of sleep disorders who recommended removal of his tonsils as well as using CPAP at bedtime. Carl returned for a cleaning recently and looked very healthy and relaxed. He reported sleeping well and going off of his blood pressure medication. He now plans to see an orthodontist to improve his bite and his smile.*

There is a strong correlation between periodontal disease and sleep apnea. Periodontal disease negatively affects cardiovascular health, promoting atherosclerosis, which is highly associated with sleep apnea. Also, severe gum disease often leads to tooth loss which may limit therapy choices for sleep apnea, like use of certain oral devices which help move the mandible forward to help with the airway (mandibular advancement devices). Future research is in progress to determine if treating periodontal disease will treat sleep apnea or vice versa.

Chapter 6

PREGNANCY AND HORMONAL FACTORS IN WOMEN

When a woman becomes pregnant, she knows it is important to maintain a healthy lifestyle for her baby and herself. It is well known that changes in hormone levels have a wide range of effects on women's bodies during pregnancy, including nausea and swelling. Less well known is the impact that hormones have on dental health during pregnancy.

We know now that high concentrations of hormones may allow aggressive bacteria to grow and cause gum disease during pregnancy unless we take good care of our gums and teeth. Uncontrolled, severe gum disease during pregnancy can create a strong immune response, which will cause inflammation and increase the risk of disease spreading throughout the body.

The relationship between high-risk pregnancies and gum disease has been studied extensively over the past ten years because gum infection has been found to be very common among women in this group. Some studies have reported that up to 40 percent of pregnant women have some form of gum disease, and the rate is higher among racial and ethnic minorities and women of low socioeconomic status.

Of all pregnancies, six to eight percent are considered high risk and can result in the death of both the mother and child. Even though we have improved prenatal care through research and better technology, research continues in ways to reduce risks during pregnancy.

The American Academy of Periodontology (AAP) and the European Federation of Periodontology (EFP) urge pregnant women to maintain tooth and gum health. There is research indicating that women with gum disease may have a higher risk of giving birth to premature or low-birth-weight babies, developing preeclampsia, and suffering a miscarriage.

Premature Birth and Gum Disease

Premature birth is defined as delivery at less than 37 weeks. Premature births account for up to 10 percent of all births in the United States and are the leading cause of infant death. Prematurity has also been identified as a major risk factor for long-term neurological problems. Before the 1990s, the risk of premature birth was thought to be associated with extremes of maternal age, race, socioeconomic status, and various diseases. However, groundbreaking research in the early 1990s found evidence of a connection between maternal vaginal infection—particularly bacterial infections—and premature birth. Two major ways that untreated gum disease in the mother may impact the fetus have been identified. Mouth bacteria may directly enter the womb through the bloodstream, or the mouth bacteria may produce inflammatory toxins that reach the fetus and cause problems.

Dr. Steven Offenbacher led extensive research on gum disease and pregnancy. His findings suggest that gum infection is a risk factor for premature, low-weight births. His data shows that women with untreated moderate-to-severe gum disease have a seven times higher risk of giving birth to premature, low-weight babies.

Only non-surgical periodontal treatment is recommended during pregnancy as surgery could put too much stress on both the mother and baby. However, another study by the same group found while non-surgical treatment will reduce bacteria and inflammation, it will not eliminate the bacteria in the gums. Therefore, the best recommendation is to prevent gum disease or treat existing gum disease before pregnancy.

Research in the past three decades has reaffirmed the 1990s findings, although the exact role of gum disease in premature births is still being researched.

Preeclampsia and Gum Disease

Preeclampsia is high blood pressure during pregnancy in women whose blood pressure had been normal before pregnancy. This condition can cause organ damage, most often to the liver and kidneys. Early-onset preeclampsia may begin around 20 weeks and is a unique disorder associated with a problem in the placenta, while late-onset preeclampsia begins around 34 weeks and is usually associated with a normal placenta.

Uncontrolled, severe gum disease in women during pregnancy has been connected to an increased risk of preeclampsia. Although the factors associated with this connection are not yet understood, a study conducted on pregnant women at the time of delivery found that pregnant women with untreated severe gum disease had twice the risk for developing preeclampsia than pregnant women without severe gum disease.

> *Susie was in the first trimester of her first pregnancy when she came to our office. She was in her early 30s and told us during the examination that she did not receive regular dental care. She came to us because she noticed her gums were enlarged and bled easily. After our examination, we explained to her that she had severe gum disease. We recommended non-surgical deep cleaning as the initial phase of treatment to reduce the bacteria and inflammation. We scheduled*

her treatment for the end of her first trimester. Due to the deep pockets and severity of Susie's gum disease, we also planned surgical treatment after her baby was born.

Susie did not return for treatment until two years later. She told us that she had developed preeclampsia during her pregnancy and had almost died during the delivery of her baby. She was grateful that both she and her baby were alive and healthy. She said she remembered me telling her about the effects of severe gum disease on pregnancy, including the potential for developing preeclampsia. She wanted periodontal treatment to make sure she was healthy for any future pregnancies. Even though her experience ultimately made her too afraid to get pregnant again, she completed her periodontal treatment and has been healthy and stable since then.

Gum disease has a tremendous impact on peoples' lives. It limits lifestyles, and in Susie's case, threatened her young life and changed her future plans. If you or someone you love is thinking about getting pregnant or is already pregnant, schedule an appointment for a dental cleaning and evaluation. If you are diagnosed with gum disease, make sure you see a periodontist to get it under control before trying to get pregnant and then get regular cleanings to maintain the good oral health. Also discuss the risks with your doctor and make sure that your blood pressure is closely monitored throughout your pregnancy.

Small Infants and Gum Disease

Research on the impact of gum disease and pregnancy shows that the fetuses of women with untreated moderate-to-severe gum disease are twice as likely to measure smaller than normal in early pregnancy and that this may continue throughout the pregnancy. Some studies suggest that the risk of delivering a small infant is 11 times higher in patients with uncontrolled, severe gum disease in comparison to those without gum disease. Women with moderate to severe gum disease and high C-reactive protein (CRP) levels in their blood also have a very high risk of delivering small infants.

Gestational Diabetes and Gum Disease

Gestational diabetes is diabetes diagnosed for the first-time during pregnancy (gestation). Like other types of diabetes, gestational diabetes affects how your cells use sugar (glucose). The disease affects approximately seven percent of pregnant women and causes high blood sugar that may complicate the pregnancy and affect the overall health of the baby. Gestational diabetes is a significant cause of maternal and infant death and can result in larger babies and blood pressure issues for mothers.

Severe gum disease can cause infection and inflammation that affects the entire body. Some research has indicated that gum infection may increase insulin resistance during pregnancy. That resistance can cause blood sugars to spike and result in gestational diabetes.

> *Ann was referred to us for the treatment of bleeding gums. She was 36 years old and pregnant, and she had just been diagnosed with gestational diabetes. We worked with her to improve her periodontal health using non-surgical periodontal treatment.*
>
> *Ann was very motivated to do anything to have a healthy baby, and she worked closely with us and her physician. With a healthy diet and lifestyle changes, as well as good dental hygiene and regular dental cleanings, she was able to control her gestational diabetes and deliver a healthy baby boy. She has been seeing us faithfully every three months for a professional dental cleaning. We have educated her on the possibility of developing type 2 diabetes later in life and the importance of a healthy lifestyle and excellent oral health to prevent chronic disease.*

While any pregnancy complication is concerning, there is good news if you or a loved one are considering becoming pregnant. Expectant mothers can help control gestational diabetes by eating healthy foods and exercising. Professional dental cleanings and good oral hygiene are critical in preventing any periodontal issues as well. In more serious cases, medications can help control gestational diabetes. Controlling blood sugar can keep you and your baby healthy and prevent a difficult delivery.

Pregnancy Tumors

Sometimes a large lump with deep red pinpoint markings forms on inflamed gum tissue during pregnancy. The lump glistens and may bleed and crust over. These growths are called pregnancy tumors and can occur at any time during pregnancy, though they most often develop during the second or third trimester. They are usually painless but can sometimes cause discomfort and make eating and speaking difficult.

Pregnancy tumors are not cancerous and cannot be spread to others. A pregnancy tumor is an extreme inflammatory reaction to a high level of hormones and a local irritation to the gums caused by food particles or plaque stuck in between the teeth and gums. The tumors occur in up to ten percent of pregnant women and are more common in women with gingivitis.

Most pregnancy tumors reduce in size or even disappear after delivery. In extreme cases, if the tumor is interfering with speech or eating, it can be surgically removed.

How Does Gum Disease Affect Pregnant Women?

There is evidence that bacteria and inflammatory toxins caused by gum disease can get into the bloodstream and spread throughout the body. During pregnancy, the fetus may be exposed to mouth bacteria, toxins, or other inflammatory substances through the blood vessels that provide oxygen-rich blood to the placenta. This could cause a series of events that may result in preeclampsia, prematurity, low-weight birth, smaller babies, or miscarriage.

All research points to a connection between increased hormone activity and impacts from uncontrolled severe gum disease. Severe gum disease may increase CRP levels, and as an inflammatory substance, this could potentially be the connection between uncontrolled severe gum disease and high-risk pregnancies. Some studies have shown that antibodies of certain bacteria related to gum disease were elevated in women who had suffered miscarriages.

Fluctuations in hormones during the menstrual cycle have also been shown to affect gum disease, with women reporting increased inflammation and discomfort. In addition, research indicates a connection between the use of oral contraceptives and increased inflammation in patients with gum disease.

Treatment and Prevention

The best way to manage risks caused by hormones and gum disease is to protect the health of your teeth and gums.

- Visit your dentist/periodontist and get checked and treated for gum disease before planning your pregnancy.
- Brush your teeth carefully twice a day for two minutes with a toothpaste.
    - Ask your dentist to show you a good brushing method to remove plaque.
    - Brushing is best with a small-headed toothbrush with soft filaments. Make sure it is comfortable to hold.
- Floss at least once a day to remove debris between your teeth. This will help to prevent the buildup of plaque.
- Avoid sugary drinks (soft drinks, sweet tea, etc.) and do not indulge in sugary foods too often. Try to keep them to mealtimes.
- If you are hungry between meals, snack on foods such as vegetables, fresh fruit, or plain yogurt, and avoid foods high in sugar or acid.
- Use an antibacterial mouthwash regularly. Avoid mouthwashes that contain alcohol.
- Stop smoking. It can make gum disease worse.

- A daily salt rinse (one teaspoon of salt added to a cup of warm water) can help reduce gum inflammation. Swirl the wash around your mouth a few times before spitting it out (do not swallow it).
- If you have vomiting, rinse your mouth with plain water after each time you are sick. This will help prevent the acid in the vomit from damaging your teeth.
    - Do not brush your teeth straight away because they will be softened by the acid from your stomach. Instead, wait about an hour before brushing.

Dental Treatment During Pregnancy

It is important to emphasize that all preventive dental treatment procedures are safe throughout pregnancy, and these, combined with good oral hygiene, are usually effective in preventing gum disease and maintaining oral health. However, general obstetric guidelines recommend avoiding all major dental treatment (unless the patient is in pain) during the first trimester due to possible stress to the fetus.

What to expect during your dental visit:

A dental healthcare professional evaluating a woman of childbearing age will ask whether they are currently pregnant or trying to become pregnant. If the answer is *yes*, the dental healthcare professional will consider the pregnancy before beginning dental treatment. A comprehensive medical history review will be conducted to rule out diabetes and heart disease. Blood pressure will be checked for signs of hypertension.

If the patient has healthy teeth and gums, the treatment will focus on gum disease prevention to protect both mother and child. They will discuss common problems that may occur during pregnancy, including increased bleeding or enlarged gums. The dental healthcare professional will stress the importance of maintaining good oral hygiene and regular dental cleanings throughout the pregnancy. However, if more serious issues are present, the dental healthcare professional will take further steps, including:

1. Pregnancy and Gingivitis

   If the patient is diagnosed with gingivitis, treatment will focus on reducing bacteria and inflammation with thorough and meticulous dental cleanings. Regular dental appointments will be scheduled to help maintain oral health. The dental healthcare professional will continue to assess the patient for high blood pressure, diabetes, and heart disease during each visit and continuously stress the importance of proper oral hygiene.

2. Pregnancy and Gum disease (Periodontitis)

   The professional treatment of gum disease during pregnancy is usually non-surgical and usually involves deep cleanings to reduce bacteria and inflammation. Excessive trauma should be avoided to prevent stress to the baby. The surgical removal of any local gum enlargements (pregnancy tumors) is usually delayed, if possible, until after the delivery of the baby. If the pregnancy tumor is too large and is interfering with eating, talking, or appearance, it can be removed in the second or third trimester. The dental healthcare professional will continue to assess the patient for high blood pressure, diabetes, and heart disease during each visit and continuously stress the importance of proper oral hygiene.

Any women of child bearing age are recommended to inform their medical professional of any dental issues. Preventative dental care is recommended if they are planning to get pregnant. Many of these serious issues can be reduced easily with professional dental care.

Chapter 7

GUM DISEASE AND THE GUT

Gut Dysbiosis, Cancer, Obesity and Metabolic Syndrome

You may have heard someone refer to their abdomen as their "gut," but that is not completely accurate. The gut, also known as the digestive tract or gastrointestinal (GI) tract, is the tube that connects the mouth to the rectum. Everything you eat and drink moves through the gut. Nutrients from the food you eat will eventually travel through the cells that line the gut and enter your bloodstream. Everything else is waste and will continue through the tube to the rectum. However, if toxic substances enter your gut, they can leak into your body. This can cause big problems because whatever happens within your gut from beginning to end can affect your entire body.

Living inside your gut are about 300-500 different kinds of bacteria containing nearly two million genes. Paired with other tiny organisms like viruses and fungi, they make up what is known as the gut microbiome. The good bacteria that live in the gut microbiome help with digestion. They also keep the bad bacteria under control by multiplying so often that the bad bacteria do not have enough space to grow. When you have this healthy balance of bacteria in your gut, it is in a healthy state of equilibrium. This equilibrium helps keep the protective barrier in the digestive tract intact and prevents toxins from escaping through the gut lining and into the bloodstream where they have the perfect travel system to move throughout the body causing problems.

Studies suggest that gut bacteria in healthy people are different from bacteria in people with certain diseases. People who are sick may have too little or too much of a certain type of bacteria—or they may lack a wide variety of bacteria—and, while some gut bacteria may help protect our bodies from illness, others may increase our risk. A strong connection has been found between bacteria in the gut and several chronic diseases.

How the Mouth Can Affect the Gut

We know that mouth bacteria can enter the bloodstream and spread throughout the body. We also know that mouth bacteria have been associated with a variety of systemic diseases. The most common way for mouth bacteria to enter the gut is through swallowed saliva, nutrients, and drinks. Research has shown high levels of mouth bacteria in the guts of patients suffering from chronic diseases.

For patients with mouth issues like tooth decay, cavities, or gum disease, swallowing the bad bacteria associated with these problems can result in gut dysbiosis. Dysbiosis is an imbalance in the gut microbiome in which the bad bacteria overwhelm the good bacteria. The resulting inflammation caused by the bacteria could lead to a breakdown in the gut's barrier protection and allow toxins from the gut to seep into the body. This is how a leaky gut develops. Many types of bad bacteria swallowed in saliva are destroyed by the acid in our stomachs. However, P. Gingivalis, one of the most aggressive mouth bacteria, is acid resistant; therefore, it is a major culprit in the development of a leaky gut. Leaky gut triggers the immune system, causes digestive problems and inflammation, and allows bacteria, toxins, and other inflammatory substances to break through the cells lining the gut (the gut barrier) and enter the bloodstream.

Leaky gut is a contributing factor in other chronic diseases such as inflammatory bowel disease (IBD), HIV infection, liver cirrhosis, colon cancer, primary acid reflux disease, and alcoholism. IBD, which includes Crohn's disease and ulcerative colitis, is defined as "chronic inflammation of the gastrointestinal tract." The Centers for Disease Control and Prevention estimates that about three million Americans were diagnosed with IBD in 2015, the last year a study of this magnitude was undertaken. The risk of developing leaky gut is particularly high for people with uncontrolled, severe gum disease because without diligent treatment they will ingest high levels of P. Gingivalis over a long period of time. Common signs of leaky gut are indigestion, stomach pain, cramps, nausea, vomiting, diarrhea, body aches, and/or an increase in bowel movements. These symptoms could happen for a variety of reasons, but if you are persistently experiencing any of them, talk to your doctor.

How the Gut Can Affect the Mouth

Anything that causes an overgrowth of unhealthy bacteria in the gut can also increase the growth of bad bacteria in the mouth. When the gut microbiome becomes unbalanced, causing a leaky gut and inflammation, the immune system becomes compromised. This can impact the entire body, including the microbiome of bacteria in the mouth. When the microbiome in the mouth becomes unbalanced, bad bacteria increases in the dental plaque, the sticky white substance that forms around the teeth and gums. Unhealthy dental plaque is the culprit that causes tooth decay and gum disease.

As bad bacteria increase, they can cause infection in the gum tissues around the teeth and decay in the tooth surfaces. The infection can then pass through the gum spaces surrounding the teeth and leak into the bloodstream just as gut infections can pass through the gut lining into the bloodstream. The result of "leaky gum tissues" may be the same as a "leaky gut." Both may cause chronic inflammation that leads to chronic diseases throughout the body. Chronic diseases commonly associated with gum disease and leaky gut include cancer, obesity, diabetes, atherosclerosis, and rheumatoid arthritis.

Stomach and Throat Cancer

Stomach cancer is one of the most common chronic diseases worldwide. More than 20 thousand new cases are diagnosed and more than 10 thousand people die from the disease in the United States each year. We know that *H. Pylori* bacteria growing in the stomach cause stomach cancer and that cigarette smoking and eating high levels of salt and preserved foods increase the risk of developing stomach cancer. There is also an increasing amount of evidence that certain mouth bacteria can contribute to both mouth and gut cancers. For example, P. Gingivalis has been found in precancerous stomach and colon cancer lesions.

Because gum disease is a chronic, destructive disease in the mouth, it is believed that a group of mouth bacteria is responsible for causing infections that lead to chronic inflammation throughout the body. A connection has been found between the bacteria in saliva and stomach cancer in individuals with gum disease.

P. Gingivalis and other gum disease-producing bacteria have also been linked to throat cancer. An imbalance of salivary bacteria has been found in patients with mouth and throat cancer. Although more research is needed, studies suggest that exposure to toxins in the cells causes the cells to grow and turn cancerous. Increased bacteria due to severe gum inflammation may be an important contributing factor for a higher risk of developing cancer. Based on these new studies, severe gum disease treatment and the prevention of gum infections are needed as strategies for preventing stomach cancer.

> *Chang was a 60-year-old patient who came to our office with severe gum disease and a history of smoking, alcoholism, and chewing tobacco. Counseling—to help him give up smoking and control his other unhealthy habits—was not very successful. He was also not practicing good dental hygiene, so his gum disease was getting worse.*
>
> *One day, during a routine cleaning, the hygienist discovered a hard, grayish-white ulcer on the side of his tongue. Chang said that it had been there a while, so we recommended a biopsy. At first, he told us that he would come back at a later date to do the biopsy, but at my urging, he consented. We numbed him, removed the ulcer with a laser, and sent it to the lab. Lasers are especially useful in reducing bleeding during tongue surgeries. The results came back positive for squamous cell carcinoma. This cancer is commonly seen on the side of the tongue and is usually associated*

with smoking or chewing tobacco. We referred Chang to an oncologist for treatment. This was aggressive cancer that was caught and treated early and contained with surgical intervention, and Chang was grateful. The surgery was a wake-up call for Chang to control his health and quit his destructive habits.

Obesity

According to the World Health Organization (WHO), obesity is defined as an excessive accumulation of fat that may impair health. An adult is considered overweight if their body mass index (BMI) is over 25 and obese if their BMI is over 30. The prevalence of overweight and obese adults has increased worldwide during the last few decades, raising concerns about health and socioeconomic impacts. Obesity is accompanied by a state of low-grade inflammation and is a contributing factor in major chronic diseases such as cardiovascular disease, diabetes, and potentially gum disease.

Gum disease and obesity are among the most common chronic disorders affecting the world's populations, and recent studies suggest a potential link between being overweight, or obese, and gum disease.

Obesity-related inflammation may promote gum disease by increasing inflammation in the mouth and promoting increased bad bacteria on the tooth root surface. However, gum disease also produces inflammatory toxins that may promote obesity and other chronic metabolic diseases. The exact connection between obesity and gum disease has yet to be established. However, fatty tissue actively secretes a variety of toxins and hormones that contribute to inflammation. This points to a connection between obesity, gum disease, and other related inflammatory diseases.

The waist-to-hip ratio in overweight and obese adults has also been associated with a higher risk of tooth loss. However, the results suggest that markers of inflammation such as C-reactive protein (CRP) may be the reason for the association between obesity and tooth loss in men.

Another study concluded that being overweight, obese, gaining weight, and increasing waist circumference may be risk factors for the development of gum disease or the advancement of existing gum disease.

Metabolic Syndrome

Metabolic syndrome is a group of disorders including abdominal obesity, high blood pressure, insulin resistance, etc., associated with an increased risk of diabetes and cardiovascular events. The suspected link between metabolic syndrome and gum disease may be related to increased levels of inflammatory toxins, abdominal fat, and high blood sugar. Common risk factors for metabolic syndrome include smoking, unhealthy diet, and low socioeconomic status.

> *Stanley was a 55-year-old patient referred to us for severe gum disease. He had bleeding gums, pus, and*

abscesses in several teeth. He also had a history of diabetes and high blood pressure, and he was overweight. When I see a patient with these classic signs, I usually tell them that we must work to improve all the issues, not just treat the gum disease.

Our plan for Stanley's initial gum treatment was to remove all the irritants and reduce the infection. At the same time, we recommended nutritional counseling to help with his gut issues. The nutritionist advised Stanley to start probiotics and supplements. He was also placed on an anti-inflammatory diet—mainly avoiding refined sugars, white flour, alcohol, and caffeine. Stanley worked closely with his medical doctor and added a daily walk to his regimen.

The change in Stanley over the next few months was miraculous. He lost weight, and his blood sugar levels and blood pressure were well controlled. We also treated and controlled Stanley's gum disease with gum surgery and saved his teeth, improving his health and happiness.

Treatment and Prevention

Several factors impact both gum disease and leaky gut, including:

- Lifestyle habits
- Oral hygiene

- Dietary habits
- Smoking
- Genetics
- Salivary gland dysfunction

Treatment for chronic diseases in patients with severe gum disease and a leaky gut must include healing the gut, the mouth, and any other source of infection. The balance of bacteria in the body must be restored to a healthy state. This healing process will support the overall immune system.

Make Good Lifestyle Choices

The first and most important action to take is to stop whatever is causing unhealthy changes in the gut and damage to the gut lining. Poor lifestyle choices, which could cause disease and prevent healing, need to be identified. Specifically, exercise, sleep, and stress need to be evaluated and corrected, as necessary. The best treatment is prevention, so take good care of your total body health:

- If you smoke, stop
- If you do not exercise, start
    - Work with your doctor to create a smoking cessation program and an exercise program based on your health needs
- Get seven to eight hours of sleep each night
- Practice stress reduction techniques

- Make sure that you are getting the right nutrients and vitamins
    - Talk to your doctor about any vitamins and supplements you may need

All these efforts and lifestyle changes could prevent chronic disease. They might also improve your condition if you are already living with a chronic disease.

Practice Good Oral Hygiene

Good oral hygiene to prevent gum disease and periodontal therapy to control existing gum disease may help reduce the risk of developing leaky gut and other digestive disorders. Poor mouth hygiene that results in severe gum disease has been identified as a factor in the development of leaky gut; therefore, brushing your teeth at least twice per day, regular flossing, rinsing with mouthwash, and regular professional cleanings will go a long way toward keeping your body healthy.

Regular Medical and Dental Visits

If you have been diagnosed with gum disease and leaky gut, treatment to remove existing infection and regular periodontal cleanings to prevent future infections are necessary to control bad bacteria and keep it from continuing to enter the gut. For mild to moderate gum disease, routine scaling and root planing to remove the bacteria will assist the body in healing. In advanced cases, periodontal surgery may be helpful to reduce infection and save your teeth. Whatever periodontal treatment is required must include proper techniques for the daily care of teeth and gums and regular periodontal cleanings. It is also important to talk about these problems with your medical professional for overall health.

Eat Healthy, Wholesome Food

Nutrient-dense, anti-inflammatory foods will help bring the gut microbiome into a state of balance as well as assist in the healing of the gut lining. Studies have shown that a healthy diet can also significantly reduce gingivitis by reducing inflammation. Remember that gingivitis is the first type of gum disease that appears, and it is the only curable type of gum disease. A diet low in carbohydrates, rich in Omega-3 fatty acids, rich in vitamins C and D, and rich in fiber has shown to reduce inflammation in the mouth; therefore, your diet and good management of your gut microbiome are part of the equation for the good health of your teeth, gums, and total body. Foods that help reduce inflammation include:

- Fruit and berries - blackberries, cherries, raspberries, citrus fruit, apples
- Fermented and cultured foods - yogurt, milk kefir, sauerkraut, kimchi
- Whole grains - oats, barley, whole wheat, rye

- Vegetables and herbs - garlic, onions, mushrooms, spinach, spices, herbs, cabbage, broccoli, kale
- Seafood and freshwater fish

Note: People who are allergic to gluten or have a sensitivity to it may have an inflammatory reaction to grains such as wheat, rye, barley, etc.

Foods with added sugars and processed carbohydrates promote inflammation, encourage the growth of bad bacteria in the mouth, and aggravate leaky guts. Avoid these foods:

- Desserts and drinks with refined sugar, candy, cakes, cookies, and soft drinks
- Foods fried in corn oil, safflower oil, and other processed oils

Good bacteria are picky eaters, and they much prefer plant-based foods. To support and protect the good bacteria in your body so they can do their job and protect your health, establish a nutrient-dense, anti-inflammatory diet. Talk to your doctor or a nutritionist about helping you establish a healthy diet specific to your needs. Eating wholesome foods will benefit your gut microbiome, your teeth, and your gums.

The Role of Prebiotics and Probiotics

A recent study described how prebiotics and probiotics help balance the gut microbiome and suggested that they may also help with the prevention and treatment of cardiovascular disease. The study found low-grade inflammation caused by the immune system fighting toxins released into the bloodstream due to leaky gut.

Prebiotics are food substances that help nourish the bacteria living within the gut. You can find prebiotics in foods like onions, garlic, Jerusalem artichokes, bananas, asparagus, jicama, and chicory root. Prebiotics cannot be digested by your body, so they hang out in the gut. They are the preferred food source for good probiotic bacteria and help promote their growth throughout the gut. Prebiotics keep probiotic bacteria happy and healthy, encouraging them to stick around.

Probiotics are the "good bacteria" that can provide numerous health benefits, including supporting your digestive and immune health. You can incorporate probiotics into your day with supplements or foods like yogurt, kimchi, and sauerkraut.

Future Treatment Options

Very recently, Fusobacterium nucleatum—a bacterium that resides in the mouth—has been strongly linked to the progression and spread of cancer, or metastasis of some cancers like colon, pancreas, throat, and possibly breast. Research indicates that the bacterium travels through the blood, infects tumor cells, and creates an immune response known to cause cancer cells to migrate. The infection causes dramatic inflammation as we have seen in so many other diseases, and the inflammation is a major contributor to the metastasis. Some scientists believe that Fusobacterium nucleatum could be used to carry cancer drugs straight to the cancer cells for targeted treatment.

A Healthy Outcome

We have plenty of evidence that gum disease and leaky gut are connected to many chronic diseases, including stomach cancer, throat cancer, obesity, and metabolic syndrome. Unhealthy gums and an unhealthy gut put the entire body at risk, and the mouth-gut connection affects the entire body. Protecting the healthy bacteria that grow in our bodies is critical for our overall health.

To obtain the best health in your mouth and gut, you should:

- Make good lifestyle choices
- Practice good oral hygiene
- Eat nutrient-dense, anti-inflammatory foods
- Repopulate the healthy bacteria in your gut
- Feed the healthy bacteria in your gut the fiber they need to thrive
- Regular visits to your dentist/periodontist as well as medical professionals

Chapter 8

GUM DISEASE AND THE BRAIN

Alzheimer's Disease, Autism Spectrum Disorder (ASD)

There is much more that we need to understand about treatments for brain disorders such as Alzheimer's and autism. However, there is new and emerging information that shows a connection between these disorders and gum disease.

Alzheimer's and Other Diseases

As proffered in previous chapters, gum disease affects almost every system in the body. Earlier in the book, I stated that P. Gingivalis, one of the most aggressive types of mouth bacteria, have been found in the brain. Antibodies to P. Gingivalis have also been found in the brain. Doctors and scientists once believed that substances like bacteria and antibodies could not reach the brain because they could not get past the blood-brain barrier, but these discoveries are proof that the blood-brain barrier can be breached. In the past five years, several studies have found potential connections between gum disease and Alzheimer's.

Alzheimer's is the most common cause of dementia, a general term for the loss of memory and other cognitive abilities serious enough to interfere with daily life. Between 60 to 80 percent of dementia patients are diagnosed with Alzheimer's.

The greatest known risk factor for developing Alzheimer's is increasing age, with the majority of patients 65 and older. However, Alzheimer's is not a normal part of aging and is not even specific to old age. A less known statistic shows that approximately 200 thousand Americans under the age of 65 have younger-onset Alzheimer's disease, also known as early-onset Alzheimer's.

Alzheimer's is a progressive disease in which dementia symptoms gradually and tragically worsen over a number of years. In its early stages, memory loss is mild, but with late-stage Alzheimer's, individuals lose the ability to carry on a conversation and respond to their environment. The disease is the sixth leading cause of death in the United States.

Although we still think that the brain may be more well protected than other organs, some studies have focused on the fact that localized inflammation is clearly evident in several neurological disorders. More studies are needed to understand the impact of inflammation on the brain; however, remember that when bad bacteria like P. Gingivalis attack a certain part of the body, the immune system wages war on the intruders. It sends in antibodies, and the antibodies create inflammation as a way to protect the body. However, if the antibodies cannot defeat the bacteria quickly, both the antibodies and bacteria continue to multiply, causing dangerous, prolonged inflammation and the destruction of the surrounding tissue. Now, imagine this destructive process taking place in the fragile tissue of the brain.

Although we currently have more questions than answers in this area, recent studies identified P. Gingivalis in autopsy specimens from the brains of people who had Alzheimer's disease. Bacteria were present in the brain fluid as well as the saliva of individuals with mild-to-moderate Alzheimer's.

Research released earlier this year revealed that older adults with signs of gum disease and mouth infections at the beginning of the study were more likely to develop Alzheimer's during the study period. Among those 65 years or older, both Alzheimer's diagnoses and deaths were associated with antibodies to fight P. Gingivalis, which can cluster with other bacteria and increase the risks. Infections in the mouth preceded the diagnosis of dementia. It is also possible that patients with dementia have difficulty brushing and flossing effectively, which in turn increases the likelihood of infections and gum disease. The research showed a potential association between gum disease and Alzheimer's, but it did not discover the cause. More studies are needed to test whether treating infections where P. Gingivalis is present can reduce the development of or existing symptoms of dementia.

A recent report published in *Science Advances* also found a connection between P. Gingivalis and Alzheimer's. The researchers analyzed brain tissue, the fluid surrounding the brain, and saliva from Alzheimer's patients, both living and deceased. Gingipains, toxins secreted by P. Gingivalis, were found in 96 percent of the brain tissue samples examined. The highest levels were in patients with symptoms of Alzheimer's disease. Another study found that P. Gingivalis suppresses the immune response, which may suggest an increased risk for disease in patients at risk for Alzheimer's.

The recent discovery that bacteria and antibodies can move through the blood-brain barrier, as well as the evidence of a connection between P. Gingivalis and Alzheimer's, is opening up new avenues in the research of this dreadful disease. We hope that with continued analysis, better treatment options will emerge. One fact has already become evident—the epidemic of gum disease is impacting our health more than we ever imagined, highlighting a greater need for prevention and early treatment.

Treatment and Prevention

While there is currently no cure for Alzheimer's disease or a way to stop or slow its progression, there are drug and non-drug options that may help treat symptoms. Understanding available options can help patients and their caretakers cope with symptoms and improve the patient's quality of life. These drug and non-drug options can provide people with comfort, dignity, and independence for a longer period of time and can encourage and assist their caregivers as well.

> *Lawrence is an Alzheimer's patient I have been treating for some time. On his first visit, his mouth was in pretty bad shape. He had severe gum disease and missing teeth, and he could not eat very well. He had a lower partial denture which he kept misplacing. We selected a course of treatment to get his gum disease under control and improve his quality of life. His upper teeth were treated with gum surgery and were returned to a healthy and functional state. However, the few remaining bottom teeth were severely infected and needed to be removed. We placed implants and delivered a full set of lower fixed implant-supported teeth in collaboration with his regular dentist.*
>
> *We believe we improved the quality of Lawrence's life by eliminating the inflammation and disease in his mouth. This helped him eat better with his healthy*

upper teeth and the lower dental implant-supported fixed teeth. Based on emerging science and research, treating Lawrence's gum disease should have a positive impact on his Alzheimer's disease progression. He can now eat a healthy diet, and he is very happy. Improving his condition has also helped his wife, who is Lawrence's main caregiver. She now has a husband who eats well and does not keep losing his dentures.

Research conducted on mice showed that P. Gingivalis could spread to the brain and caused neurons to be destroyed and reproduced the symptoms of Alzheimer's. In response to this study, some companies are developing investigational drugs to reduce inflammation and the destruction of neurons in the brain as a result of P. Gingivalis bacteria. Other studies are focusing on creating targeted treatment options to destroy gingipains as opposed to using antibiotics, which kill both good and bad bacteria. If any of these treatments prove successful, there may be opportunities for their use beyond the Alzheimer's patient.

Lifestyle changes such as a healthy diet, exercise, reducing inflammation, and treating gum disease may help prevent or slow down this disease.

Prevention and treatment of gum disease may be a promising and easy way to reduce the risk of Alzheimer's in high-risk individuals. The American Academy of Periodontology encourages older adults and other at-risk individuals to maintain good dental care and promptly treat gum disease to help mitigate Alzheimer's risk. Routine brushing, flossing once a day, and visiting a periodontist can help identify gum disease and provide treatment as needed, potentially diminishing the risk of developing Alzheimer's.

Autism Spectrum Disorder (ASD)

Children with autism spectrum disorder are often restricted, rigid, and even obsessive in their behaviors, activities, and interests. Symptoms may include:

- Repetitive body movements (hand flapping, rocking, and spinning)
- Moving constantly
- Obsessive attachment to unusual objects (rubber bands, keys, light switches)

Autism specifically affects brain function for communication and social interaction skills. In fact, the primary symptom of autism is a lack of communication skills. Autistic children also have problems with language, behavior, and social skills. Early diagnosis, early intensive remedial education, and behavioral therapy are proven techniques to improve the social skills of an autistic child.

Children with autism are likely to develop teeth and gum problems for a number of reasons such as unusual dental habits, medications, and poor food choices. Difficult behaviors, such as head banging, picking at the lips, and chewing on harmful objects like stones, can also contribute to dental problems. Autistic children also prefer soft foods that they tend to pouch at the back of their mouths for long periods of time.

An imbalance between the good and bad bacteria in the gut is emerging as one of the causes of autism. There is evidence to suggest that the gut microbiome can influence the brain by using signals to communicate. An imbalance in the gut bacteria may affect the patient's emotions, anxiety level, social behaviors, and brain development. Gut problems are common in children with autism and can include constipation, diarrhea, bloating, abdominal pain, reflux, vomiting, etc.

Autistic children with severe gum disease can swallow thousands of bacteria that then go into the gut and cause dysbiosis, eventually leading to leaky gut and inflammation. The bacteria that escape into the bloodstream through the gut lining could also end up in the brain if not blocked by the blood-brain barrier. Studies have shown that children with autism do not seem to have strong blood-brain barriers. Because the barrier is not as protective, the bacteria and toxins could actually go into the brain and cause inflammation of the brain and the nervous system, which may explain why autistic children often have nervous system problems. Several brain disorders have been reported, but further studies are needed to fully understand the impact of the weak blood-brain barrier in relation to autism.

Treatment

It is clear that mouth bacteria can find their way to the brain through a number of pathways, and a connection between mouth bacteria and other brain disorders has been made. As the evidence for an association between mouth bacteria and ASD rests on a few studies only, further research in this field is necessary.

Treating autism by managing healthy gut bacteria is showing promise. Oral probiotics have demonstrated positive effects on behaviors such as anxiety, depression, ASD, obsessive-compulsive disorder, and memory. Also, prebiotics play a limited role in reducing the gastrointestinal and behavioral symptoms in children with autism and, when combined with an exclusion diet (gluten and casein free), could potentially affect social behavior.

The Role of Prebiotics and Probiotics

Prebiotics and probiotics can help balance the gut microbiome. As detailed in Chapter 7, prebiotics are food substances that help nourish the bacteria living within the gut. They encourage good bacteria to grow and maintain a healthy balance. Probiotics are the "good bacteria." They provide numerous health benefits, including supporting your digestive and immune health.

In a study where bacteria-transfer therapy was combined with antibiotics, bowel cleanses, and a stomach-acid suppressant, patients with autism had significant improvements in gastrointestinal symptoms, autism-related symptoms, and gut bacteria. A follow-up on the children two years after treatment found that most improvements in symptoms were maintained.

Good oral hygiene and regular dental cleanings may help reduce bacteria and their impact on the health of ASD patients.

Other Conditions

Mouth bacteria can enter the bloodstream following even routine activities such as chewing, flossing, and brushing. This may contribute to several neurological diseases, including epileptic seizures, multiple sclerosis, migraines, and Parkinson's disease. However, more studies are needed to understand the impact of mouth bacteria on neurological diseases.

Conclusion

From all the previous and ongoing research, we know that patients with severe gum disease may have a higher chance of developing neurological conditions like Alzheimer's or autism. This raises the bar even higher to prevent gum disease and conduct more research to develop additional treatment and prevention options.

For patients and their caregivers, it is so important to keep the teeth and gums healthy:

- Brush your teeth gently twice a day with a soft-bristle brush and toothpaste.
- Clean in between your teeth with floss or an interdental brush.
- See a periodontist/dentist regularly for cleanings and treatment for any existing gum disease.

The connection between gum disease, Alzheimer's, autism, and other brain disorders is an emerging field in medical research. There is still much that we don't know, but it is promising to have simple treatment solutions based on the new research. If you know anyone with Alzheimer's or autism, encourage them to maintain good dental habits with regular checkups, and if they already have gum disease, make sure the gum disease is treated and their overall health is maintained through good lifestyle habits.

Chapter 9

SUMMARY AND PRACTICAL TIPS

As you have seen throughout the previous chapters, inflammation is the common denominator in the most prevalent, serious health conditions we face today. Preventing inflammation through maintaining healthy teeth and gums and a healthy body should be our primary goal. However, if inflammation exists due to disease, a holistic approach that identifies and simultaneously treats each condition causing the inflammation is necessary.

During the writing of this book, the COVID-19 pandemic rages on, unleashing cytokine storms that generate inflammation throughout the body and increase the chances of serious infection and death in patients who contract the disease. Reducing inflammation and thus reducing the damage of this virus is profoundly important to our individual and community health.

It is impossible to successfully control inflammation caused by disease in one part of the body if a different disease is causing inflammation in another part of the body. Your body is a whole system that works together. Therefore, if one part of your body—say, your mouth—is inflamed, over time, other parts of your body will be impacted. The bacteria causing the inflammation will not just stay in your mouth.

Inflammation, in itself, is not bad. It is part of the body's defense mechanism and is how the immune system recognizes and removes harmful and foreign toxins so it can begin the healing process. However, the key is to make sure that inflammation does not stay in your body for too long. Inflammation that continues over time because of an immune system fighting unchecked bacteria and infection causes damage that will only continue to grow.

Think of prolonged inflammation as a fire in your body that you cannot see or feel. "It's a smoldering process that injures your tissues, joints, and blood vessels, and you often do not notice it until significant damage is done," says Dr. Andrew Luster of the Center for Immunology and Inflammatory Diseases at Harvard-affiliated Massachusetts General Hospital. The damage might show up as arthritis, heart disease, stroke, or even Alzheimer's disease. "The goal," says Dr. Luster, "is to keep inflammation in check and not let the fire run wild." Reducing inflammation is key to getting this fire under control.

How to Reduce Inflammation

Reducing inflammation should be a foundational step in living a healthy life.

I have shared tips throughout this book on how to reduce inflammation and live a healthy life specific to the diseases in each chapter. Below is a compilation of the overall steps you can take to stay healthy and reduce inflammation in your body:

- **Fight gum disease.** If your gums bleed when you brush or floss, you most likely have inflammation. Make an appointment to see your dentist for a checkup and step up your oral hygiene. Flossing every day is so crucial that it's one of the questions included in the "Living to 100 Life Expectancy Calculator" created by Thomas Perls, Boston University. There is only one question on the quiz that addresses flossing, and the calculator estimates that this *yes* or *no* could be worth up to one year of your life.
- **Treat high cholesterol.** Get your levels tested, and, if they are deemed too high, speak with your doctor about taking statins to keep lipids under control. Help reduce cholesterol with healthy diet and exercise.
- **Quit smoking.** This is good all-around health advice. More specifically, the toxins from smoking have a direct link to inflammation.

- **Eat healthy foods:**
  - Eat more plants. Whole plant foods have the anti-inflammatory nutrients your body needs. Eat a rainbow of fruits, veggies, whole grains, and legumes.
  - Focus on antioxidants. Antioxidants help prevent, delay, or repair some types of cell and tissue damage. They are found in colorful fruits and veggies like berries, leafy greens, beets, and avocados, as well as beans and lentils, whole grains, ginger, turmeric, and green tea.
  - Get your omega-3s. Omega-3 fatty acids play a role in regulating the body's inflammatory process and could help regulate pain related to inflammation. Find these healthy fats in salmon, tuna, and mackerel, as well as smaller amounts in walnuts, pecans, ground flaxseed, and soy.
  - Eat less red meat. Red meat can be pro-inflammatory. Are you a burger lover? Aim for a realistic goal. Substitute your lunchtime beef with fish, nuts, or soy-based protein a few times a week.
  - Cut the processed stuff. Sugary cereals and drinks, deep-fried food and pastries are all pro-inflammatory culprits. They contain plenty of unhealthy fats that are linked to inflammation. Cut back or eliminate simple sugars (like soda and candy),

beverages that contain high-fructose corn syrup (like juice drinks and sports drinks), and refined carbohydrates (like white bread and pasta).

- **Maintain a healthy weight.** Being overweight increases your risk for multiple diseases; carrying excess fat around your belly is a red flag for heart disease risk. A type of fat that accumulates in the belly (called visceral fat) secretes a molecule that causes inflammation.
- **Increase activity.** Exercising for as little as 20 minutes a day can decrease inflammation. You do not have to do an intense sweat session; moderate workouts, such as fast walking, are effective.
- **Anti-inflammatory supplements.** Research suggests that certain vitamins have anti-inflammatory potential. Many of the studies were done with supplements so amounts could be accurately measured and controlled. To take advantage of the possible benefits, start by eating foods with these vitamins. Keep in mind that *more* is not always *better*. Large amounts of certain vitamins can be risky. Talk to your doctor before you take a supplement. Supplements and vitamins include, but are not limited to, vitamin A, curcumin (a component of the spice turmeric), fish oil, ginger, resveratrol, spirulina, vitamin C, zinc, green tea, frankincense, capsaicin, bromelain, flax, etc.

- **Mental stress reduction and lifestyle changes.** Another important aspect of reducing inflammation in the body is to reduce stress. The stress hormone cortisol causes similar effects as inflammatory substances produced by infection. Meditation, massage, and other relaxation techniques should be incorporated into your daily lifestyle.
- **Other recommendations:**
  - Intermittent fasting: Intermittent fasting or reducing caloric intake has been associated with reduced inflammation. It has been suggested that many people have an excess of inflammation because they eat too much and too often. In a recent study, intermittent fasting was found to reduce the inflammatory activity of monocytes, thus reducing inflammation.
  - Getting adequate sleep: Circadian rhythms regulate sleep and the immune system, which means levels of inflammation as well. Once circadian rhythms are disrupted, we are prone to more inflammation. A consistent sleep schedule prevents this disruption and, therefore, the harmful inflammation.
  - Cold water therapy or ice-cold baths have been reported to reduce inflammatory response and help recovery. Several studies in athletes have

shown faster recovery and reduced pain and inflammation after cold water therapy.

- Practicing gratitude has been found to make people happier, sleep better, and experience fewer aches and pains.

Treatment and Prevention of Gum Disease

Periodontal bacteria, especially P. Gingivalis, is one of the most common causes of persistent inflammation due to infection. Therefore, it is important to focus on the treatment and prevention of gum disease. The goal of periodontal treatment is to reduce or eliminate these bacteria so they do not cause inflammation in the mouth and the rest of the body.

Prevention of gum disease is easily accomplished with good dental hygiene and regular visits to your periodontist or dentist to get your teeth cleaned and gums examined for disease. Remember, the initial phase of gum disease, gingivitis, is reversible and can be treated with a good professional cleaning and regular brushing and flossing to remove the irritants around the gums.

Once gum disease advances beyond gingivitis, it is no longer reversible and must be treated and controlled. When gingivitis progresses to periodontitis, it results in bone loss, which reduces the tooth support causing loose teeth, bad breath, and inflammation that affects your ability to eat and smile.

- This is achieved by a deep cleaning by the hygienist, dentist, or periodontist. Severe gum disease may require surgery to eliminate bacteria deep in the gum pockets.
- Periodontal surgery has evolved over the years, and many techniques have been developed to regrow the lost bone with bone grafts, growth factors, etc. Growth factors are natural healing substances that can be collected from your blood and used to enhance healing.
- The use of lasers has allowed rapid healing with reduced pain in most cases.
- You may also be prescribed antibiotics after surgery to prevent infection and aid in healing.

Dental Implants

In very severe cases, the infected teeth can be removed and replaced with dental implants. Your periodontist can work to grow bone to place stronger implants that with proper care can last a very long time.

The implants can be placed in bone, and a tooth is attached to it that behaves like a fixed tooth. It also prevents any bone loss that usually occurs with tooth loss and supports the adjacent teeth. Dental implants commonly used are those made of titanium. However, today we have options of metal-free implants, as well, for patients who are sensitive to titanium. Dental implants have improved the quality of life for several of my patients, providing fixed replacements for a single tooth, several teeth, and even supporting dentures. In some cases, implants have helped patients get rid of their uncomfortable dentures and regain their smiles and self-confidence. With early intervention and all these choices, we believe no one should be wearing dentures these days.

Follow-up and Re-care Visits

After gum disease is treated, regular follow-ups with the dentist are important to keep the disease controlled. We recommend regular professional cleanings four times a year for patients with gum disease. Care should include an excellent oral hygiene regimen at home by brushing twice a day, flossing at least once a day, and using an antibacterial mouthwash.

Future Research and Trends

The emerging field of microbiome and how it affects the rest of the body has helped in the understanding and treatment of several diseases. Most diseases arise from an imbalance of good and bad bacteria that results in inflammation. The key is to find a way to stop or prevent the bad bacteria from overtaking the good bacteria. We now know that many drugs used to treat systemic diseases work best in the presence of beneficial bacteria.

The mouth has its own microbiome of good and bad bacteria, and we know that an overabundance of bad mouth bacteria can result in many health problems. Therefore, I believe a healthy lifestyle with excellent dental hygiene and routine dental and medical care is the key to preventing gum disease and the other serious conditions outlined in this book. More research is required to fully understand the connection between gum disease and these debilitating diseases and how to prevent them with better dental care.

Conclusion

I typically see patients with severe gum disease in my practice. The majority of these patients struggle to control their gum disease and inflammation because they have other health conditions that are either undiagnosed or uncontrolled. These patients get frustrated because they are receiving treatment for their gum disease and practicing proper oral hygiene, but the gum disease and inflammation persist. This is when I sit down with them to discuss other health issues. I explain how their health conditions, such as smoking or diabetes, are affecting their mouth and how their mouth is affecting the rest of their body. Many times, they are surprised to hear this information since they didn't realize how bacteria and inflammation spread. I usually will consult with their medical doctor. More and more physicians are becoming aware of the connection between gum disease and several serious health conditions; however, it is still not common for some physicians to discuss this connection with their patients. Therefore, it is up to patients to arm themselves with this information and work in partnership with their physician, dentist, and periodontist to holistically treat all their conditions.

A growing number of functional medicine doctors, as well as traditional physicians, are recognizing the importance of this holistic approach. Conditions like COVID-19 are also teaching us more about the importance of preventing inflammation to stop the serious effects of disease.

In treating patients with periodontal disease over the years, I have seen several patients suffer serious health issues related to it. As we have seen in the previous chapters, inflammation related to periodontal bacterial infection can have far reaching effects on the cardiovascular system, diabetic patients, in pregnancy-related complications, gut issues, Alzheimer's and autism, and respiratory problems. While there is sufficient evidence to show a strong correlation between gum disease and these conditions, more research is required to clarify the exact processes involved to help target treatment and prevention.

All these crippling diseases are a serious burden to the healthcare system and to the patients and their families. I truly believe that treating gum disease is a simple piece of the overall puzzle that can be easily taken care of. I have often seen neglect in this aspect, which prompted me to write this book to help any patient who is struggling with these issues. I sincerely hope this information helps patients work closely with their dental and medical professionals to achieve good health and happy lives.

Thank you for arming yourself with this information. I wish you health, happiness, and a beautiful healthy smile.

REFERENCES

Abariga, Samuel A., Brian W. Whitcomb. "Periodontitis and gestational diabetes mellitus. A systematic review and metanalysis." *BMC Pregnancy Childbirth*. 16(1) (2016 Nov): 344.

Abnet, Christian C., Farin Kamangar, Sanford M. Dawsey, Rachael Z. Stolzenberg-Solomon, Demetrius Albanes, Pirjo Pietinen, Jarmo Virtamo, Philip R. Taylor. "Tooth loss is associated with increased risk of gastric non-cardia adenocarcinoma in a cohort of Finnish smokers." *Scand J Gastroenterol* 40 (2005): 681–687.

Ahn, J., C.Y. Chen, R.B. Hayes. "Oral microbiome and oral and gastrointestinal cancer risk." *Cancer Causes Control*. 23(3) (2012): 399–404.

American Academy of Periodontology. "Diabetes and periodontal diseases." *J Periodontol*. 71(4) (2000 Apr): 664-78, doi: 10.1902/jop.2000.71.4.664.

American Academy of Periodontology. "What are common signs and symptoms of periodontal disease?" Retrieved December 22, 2020. https://www.perio.org/node/258.

American Academy of Periodontology. "Workshop on inflammation." *Journal of Periodontology* (2008), Retrieved December 22, 2020. https://aap.onlinelibrary.wiley.com/toc/19433670/2008/79/8S.

American Diabetes Association. "Diagnosis and classification of diabetes mellitus." *Diabetes Care* 37(Supplement 1) (2014): S81-S90.

Ananth, Cande V., Howard F. Andrews, Panos N. Papapanou, Angela M. Ward, Emilie Bruzelius, Mary Lee Conicella, David A. Albert. "History of periodontal treatment and risk for intrauterine growth restriction (IUGR)." *BMC Oral Health*. 18(1) (2018):161.

Arter, J.L., D.S. Chi, M. Girish, S.M. Fitzgerald, B. Guha, G. Krishnaswamy. "Obstructive sleep apnea, inflammation, and cardiopulmonary disease." *Front Biosci.* 1(9) (2004): 2892-900. doi: 10.2741/1445. PMID: 15353323.

Atarashi, Koji, Wataru Suda, Chengwei Luo, Takaaki Kawaguchi, Iori Motoo, Seiko Narushima, Yuya Kiguchi. "Ectopic colonization of oral bacteria in the intestine drives TH1 cell induction and inflammation." *Science*. 358(6361) (2017): 359–365.

Azarpazhooh, Amir, James L. Leake. "Systematic review of the Association between Respiratory diseases and oral health." *Journal of Periodontology*, 77(9) (September 2006): 1465-82.

Barbaresi, W.J., S.K. Katusic, R.G. Voigt. "Autism: A review of the state of the science for pediatric primary health care clinicians." *Arch Pediatr Adolesc Med*. 160 (2006): 1167-75.

Beck, J. D., J. R. Elter, G. Heiss, D. Couper, S. M. Mauriello, S. Offenbacher. "Relationship of periodontal disease to carotid artery intima-media wall thickness. The atherosclerosis risk in communities (ARIC) study." *Arterioscler Thromb Vasc Biol*. 21(11) (2001 Nov): 1816-22, doi: 10.1161/hq1101.097803.

Beck, J., R. Garcia, G. Heiss, P. S. Vokonas, S. Offenbacher. "Periodontal disease and cardiovascular disease." *J Periodontol*. 67 (1996): 1123–1137.

Beck, J.D., P.N. Papapanou, K.H. Philips, S. Offenbacher. "Periodontal medicine. 100 years of progress." *Journal of dental research*, 98 (10) (2019): 1053-1062.

Bergström, J., S Eliasson, J Dock. "A 10-year prospective study of tobacco smoking and periodontal health." *J Periodontol.* 71(8) (2000 Aug): 1338-47, doi: 10.1902/jop.2000.71.8.1338.

Beydoun, May A., Hind A. Beydoun, Sharmin Hossain, Ziad W. El-Hajj, Jordan Weiss, Alan B. Zonderman. "Clinical and bacterial markers of periodontitis and their association with incident all-cause and Alzheimer's disease dementia in a large national survey." *Journal of Alzheimer's Disease.* 75(1) (2020): 157-172. doi: 10.3233/JAD-200064.

Bobetsis, Yiorgos A., Silvana P. Barros, Steven Offenbacher. "Exploring the relationship between periodontal disease and pregnancy complications." *J Am Dent Assoc.* 137(Suppl.) (2006): 7S–13S.

Boggess, Kim A., James D. Beck, Amy P. Murtha, Kevin Moss, Steven Offenbacher. "Maternal periodontal disease in early pregnancy and risk for a small for gestational age infant." *Am J Obstet Gynecol.* 194(5) (2006 May): 1316-22.

Boggess, Kim A., Susi Lieff, Amy P. Murtha, Kevin Moss, James Beck, Steven Offenbacher. "Maternal periodontal disease is associated with an increased risk of preeclampsia." *Obstet Gynecol.* 101(2) (2003 Feb): 227-31.

Bravo Mde, L., L.D.Serpero, A. Barceló, F.Barbé, A.Agustí, D.Gozal. "Inflammatory proteins in patients with obstructive sleep apnea with and without daytime sleepiness." *Sleep Breath,* 11(3) (2007):177-85. doi: 10.1007/s11325-007-0100-7. PMID: 17279423.

Bridges, Raymond B., James W. Anderson, Stanley R. Saxe, Kevin Gregory, Susan R. Bridges. "Periodontal status of diabetic and Non-diabetic men: Effects of smoking, diabetic control and socioeconomic factors." *Journal of Periodontology* 67 (11) (1996): 1185-1192.

Buhlin, Kåre, Anders Gustafsson, A. Graham Pockley, Johan Frostegård, Björn Klinge. "Risk factors for cardiovascular disease in patients with periodontitis." *Eur Heart J.* 24(23) (2003): 2099–2107.

Bullon, P., J.M. Morillo, M.C. Ramirez-Tortosa, J.L. Quiles, H.N. Newman, M. Battino. "Metabolic syndrome, and periodontitis: Is oxidative stress a common link?" *J Dent Res* 88 (2009): 503-518.

Caton, J.G., G. Armitage, T. Berglundh, I.L.C. Chapple, S. Jepsen, K.S. Kornman, B.L. Mealey, P.N. Papapanou, M. Sanz, M.S. Tonetti. "A new classification scheme for periodontal and peri-implant diseases and conditions - Introduction and key changes from the 1999 classification." *J Clin Periodontol.* 45 Suppl 20 (2018):S1-S8, doi: 10.1111/jcpe.12935. PMID: 29926489.

Centers for Disease Control and Prevention (CDC). "Smoking-attributable mortality, years of potential life lost, and productivity losses — United States, 2000-2004." *MMWR Morb Mortal Wkly Rep* 57(45) (2008):1226-1228.

Chiu, B. "Multiple infections in carotid atherosclerotic plaques." *Am Heart J.* 138 (1999): S534–S536.

Corbella, Stefano, Silvio Taschieri, Luca Francetti, Francesca De Siena, Massimo Del Fabbro. "Periodontal disease as a risk factor for adverse pregnancy outcomes: A systematic review and meta-analysis of case controlled studies." *Odontology* 100(2) (2012): 232-40.

Costa, A.L., C.L. Yasuda, W. Shibasaki, et al. "The association between periodontal disease and seizure severity in refractory epilepsy patients." *Seizure* 23(3) (2014): 227–230.

Cotton, Meredith. "How Our Bodies Turn Food into Energy." *Kaiser Permanente*, (2020), Retrieved November 29, 2020. https://wa.kaiserpermanente.org/healthAndWellness?item=%2Fcommon%2FhealthAndWellness%2Fconditions%2Fdiabetes%2FfoodProcess.html.

Crew, K.D., A.I. Neugut. "Epidemiology of gastric cancer." *World J Gastroenterol* 12 (2006): 354-362.

Cunningham, Timothy J., Paul I. Eke, Earl S. Ford, Israel T. Agaku, Anne G. Wheaton, and Janet B. Croft. "Cigarette smoking, tooth loss, and chronic obstructive pulmonary disease: Findings from the behavioral risk Surveillance system." *J Periodontol.* 87(4) (Apr 2016): 385–394.

Daalderop, L.A., B.V. Wieland, K. Tomsin, L. Reyes, B.W. Kramer, S.F. Vanterpool, J.V. Been. "Periodontal disease and pregnancy outcomes: Overview of systematic reviews." *JDR Clin Trans Research* 3(1) (2018): 10-27.

Danenberg, A. H. (2017). *Crazy-good living!: Healthy gums, healthy gut, healthy life: Feeding your body from cradle to grave*. Salt Lake City: Elektra Press, LLC.

Danenberg, A.I. "Leaky gut and periodontal disease and all that jazz." Retrieved November 29, 2020. https://drdanenberg.com/leaky-gut-periodontal-diseaseand-all-that-jazz/.

Danenberg, A.I. *Is Your Gut Killing You? An in-depth guide on connection between the gut, the mouth, chronic disease, and how to stay healthy*. 2020, Kindle.

Danesh, John, Jeremy G. Wheeler, Gideon M. Hirschfield, Shinichi Eda, Gudny Eiriksdottir, Ann Rumley, Gordon D. O. Lowe, Mark B. Pepys, Vilmundur Gudnason. "C-reactive protein and other circulating markers of inflammation in the prediction of coronary heart disease." *N Engl J Med* 350(14) (2004): 1387–1397.

Darveau, R.P., G. Hajishengallis, M.A. Curtis. "Porphyromonas Gingivalis as a potential community activist for disease." *J Dent Res*. 91 (2012): 816-820.

de Miguel-Infante, Ana, Maria A. Martinez-Huedo, Eduardo Mora-Zamorano, Valentín Hernández-Barrera, Isabel Jiménez-Trujillo, Carmen de Burgos-Lunar, Juan Cardenas Valladolid, et al. "Periodontal disease in adults with diabetes, prevalence and risk factors. Results of an observational study." *Int J Clin Pract.* 73.3 (2018): https://doi.org/10.1111/ijcp.132.

Detke, M., D. Raha, F. Ermini, et al. "COR388, a novel gingipain inhibitor decreases fragmentation of APOE in Alzheimer's Disease central nervous system." *J of Prev of Alzheimer's Dis.* 6 (2019): S24-S25.

Dominy, S.S., C. Lynch, F. Ermini, et al. "Porphyromonas Gingivalis in Alzheimer's disease brains: evidence for disease causation and treatment with small-molecule inhibitors." *Sci Adv.* 5 (2019): eaau3333.

Ebersole, Jeffrey L., M. John Novak, Bryan S. Michalowicz, James S. Hodges, Michelle J. Steffen, James E. Ferguson, Anthony DiAngelis, William Buchanan, Dennis A. Mitchell, Panos N. Papapanou. "Systemic immune responses in pregnancy and periodontitis: Relationship to pregnancy outcomes on Obstetrics and Periodontal therapy study." *Journal of Periodontology* 80(6) (June 2009): 953–960.

Eke, Paul I., Liang Wei, Gina O. Thornton-Evans, Luisa N. Borrell, Wenche S. Borgnakke, Bruce Dye, Robert J. Genco. "Risk indicators for periodontitis in US adults: NHANES 2009 to 2012." *J Periodontal.* 87(10) (2016): 1174–1185.

Esteves Lima, Rafael Paschoal, Renata Magalhães Cyrino, Bernardo de Carvalho Dutra, Juliana Oliveira da Silveira, Carolina Castro Martins, Luis Otávio Miranda Cota, Fernando Oliveira Costa. "Association between Periodontitis and gestational diabetes mellitus: Systematic review and meta analysis." *J Periodontol.* 87(1) (2016 Jan): 48-57.

Fan, X., A.V. Alekseyenko, J. Wu, et al. "Human oral microbiome and prospective risk for pancreatic cancer: A population-based nested case-control study." *Gut.* 67(1) (2018 Jan): 120-127.

Farrokhi, V., R. Nemati, F.C. Nichols, et al. "Bacterial lipodipeptide, Lipid 654, is a microbiome-associated biomarker for multiple sclerosis." *Clin Transl Immunology* 2(11) (2013): e8.

Figueiredo, Marina Guim Otsuka Padovan, Stefanie Yaemi Takita, Bianca Maria Ramos Dourado, Helderjan de Souza Mendes, Erick Olsen Terakado, Hélio Rubens de Carvalho Nunes, Cátia Regina Branco da Fonseca. "Periodontal disease: Repercussions in pregnant woman and newborn health — A cohort study." *PLoS One*. 14(11) (2019): e0225036.

Fiorentino, M., A. Sapone, S. Senger, et al. "Blood-brain barrier and intestinal epithelial barrier alterations in autism spectrum disorders." *Mol Autism*. 29 (Nov 2016): 49.

Firatli, E. "The relationship between clinical periodontal status and insulin-dependent diabetes mellitus. Results after 5 years." *J Periodontal*. 68(2) (1997): 136–140.

Ford, Earl S., Janet B. Croft, David M. Mannino, Anne G. Wheaton, Xingyou Zhang, Wayne H. Giles. "COPD surveillance — United States, 1999-2011." *Chest* 144(1) (2013): 284–305.

Ford, Earl S., Louise B. Murphy, Olga Khavjou, Wayne H. Giles, James B. Holt, Janet B. Croft. "Total and state-specific medical and absenteeism costs of COPD among adults aged ≥ 18 years in the United States for 2010 and projections through 2020." *Chest* 147(1) (2015): 31–45.

Gami, A.S., B.J. Witt, D.E. Howard, et al. "Metabolic syndrome and risk of incident cardiovascular events and death: a systematic review and meta-analysis of longitudinal studies." *J Am Coll Cardiol*. 49 (2007): 403-414.

Gao S., S. Li, Z.Ma, et al. "Presence of Porphyromonas Gingivalis in esophagus and its association with the clinicopathological characteristics and survival in patients with esophageal cancer." *Infect Agent Cancer*. 11 (Jan 2016): 3.

Gonzalez, A., E. Hyde, N. Sangwan, et al. "Migraines are correlated with higher levels of nitrate-, nitrite-, and nitric oxide-reducing oral microbes in the American gut project cohort." *mSystems*. 1(5) (2016): pii: e00105–16.

Grenier, D., S. Roy, F. Chandad, et al. "Effect of inactivation of the Arg- and/or Lys-gingipain gene on selected virulence and physiological properties of Porphyromonas Gingivalis." *Infect Immun*. 71 (2003): 4742-4748.

Grossi, S. G., F. B. Skrepcinski, T. DeCaro, D. C. Robertson, A. W. Ho, R. G. Dunford, R. J. Genco. "Treatment of periodontal disease in diabetics reduces glycated hemoglobin." *J Periodontol*. 68(8) (1997): 713–719.

Gunaratnam, K, B. Taylor, B. Curtis, P. Cistulli. "Obstructive sleep apnoea and periodontitis: a novel association?" *Sleep Breath* 13(3) (2009): 233-9. doi: 10.1007/s11325-008-0244-0. Epub 2009 Feb 6. PMID: 19198909.

Haffajee, A. D., S. S. Socransky. "Relationship of cigarette smoking to the subgingival microbiota." *J Clin Periodontol* 28 (2001): 377–388.

Hayes C., D. Sparrow, M. Cohen, P.S. Vokonas, R.I. Garcia. "The association between alveolar bone loss and pulmonary function: The VA Dental Longitudinal Study." *Ann Periodontol* 3(1) (1998): 257–261.

Hillier, Sharon L., Robert P. Nugent, David A. Eschenbach, Marijane A. Krohn, Ronald S. Gibbs, David H. Martin, Mary Frances Cotch, et al. "Association between bacterial vaginosis and preterm delivery of a low birth weight infant." *New England Journal of Medicine*, 333 (1995): 1737-1742.

Hung, Hsin-Chia, Walter Willett, Anwar Merchant, Bernard A. Rosner, Alberto Ascherio, and Kaumudi J. Joshipura. "Oral health and peripheral arterial disease." *Circulation* 107 (2003): 1152–1157.

Ioannidou, Effie, Tannaz Malekzadeh, Anna Dongari-Bagtzoglou. "Effect of Periodontal treatment on serum C reactive protein levels: A systematic review and meta-analysis." *Journal of Periodontology* 77(10) (October 2006): 1635-42.

Iwamoto, Yoshihiro, Fusanori Nishimura, Yoshihiko Soga, Kazu Takeuchi, Mikinao Kurihara, Shogo Takashiba, Yoji Murayama. "Antimicrobial Periodontal treatment decreases C- Reactive Protein, Tumor necrosis factor alpha, but not Adiponectin in patients with chronic periodontitis." *J Periodontol.* 74(8) (2003): 1231-6, doi: 10.1902/jop.2003.74.8.1231.

Javed, Fawad, Karin Näsström, Daniel Benchimol, Mohammad Altamash, Björn Klinge, Per-Erik Engström. "Comparison of Periodontal and Socioeconomic status between subjects with Type 2 Diabetes and non-diabetic controls." *Journal of Periodontology* 78(11) (2007): 2112-9.

Johnson, Georgia K., Margaret Hill. "Cigarette smoking and the periodontal patient." *J Periodontol* 75(2) (2004): 196–209.

Jordan, S., N. Tung, M. Casanova-Acebes, C. Chang, C. Cantoni, D. Zhang, T.H. Wirtz, et al. "Dietary Intake Regulates the Circulating Inflammatory Monocyte Pool." *Cell* 22;178(5) (2019): 1102-1114.e17. doi: 10.1016/j.cell.2019.07.050. PMID: 31442403; PMCID: PMC7357241.

Joshipura, Kaumudi J., Hsin-Chia Hung, Eric B. Rimm, Walter C. Willett, and Alberto Ascherio. "Periodontal disease, tooth loss and incidence of ischemic stroke." *Stroke* 34 (2003): 47–52.

Kang, D.W., J.G. Park, Z.E. Ilhan, et al. "Reduced incidence of *Prevotella* and other fermenters in intestinal microflora of autistic children." *PLoS One*. 8(7) (2013): e68322.

Katz, Joseph, Moshe Y. Flugelman, Avishai Goldberg, Marc Heft. "Association between periodontal pockets and elevated cholesterol and low-density lipoprotein cholesterol levels." *J Periodontol.* 73 (5) (2002): 494–500.

Kealy, J., C. Greene, M. Campbell. "Blood-brain barrier regulation in psychiatric disorders." *Neurosci Lett.* 726 (2020 May): 133664.

Keirse, M.J., K. Plutzer. "Women's attitudes to and perceptions of oral health and dental care during pregnancy." *J Perinat Med.* 38(1) (2010): 3–8.

Keller, J.J., C.S. Wu, Y.H. Chen, H.C. Lin. "Association between obstructive sleep apnoea and chronic periodontitis: a population-based study." *J Clin Periodontol.* 40(2) (2013): 111-7. doi: 10.1111/jcpe.12036. Epub 2012 Dec 4. PMID: 23211028.

Keller, Amélie, Jeanett F. Rohde, Kyle Raymond, Berit L. Heitmann. "Association Between Periodontal Disease and Overweight and Obesity: A Systematic Review." *J Periodontol.* 86(6) (2015 Jun): 766-76.

Kinane, D. F. "Causation and pathogenesis of periodontal disease." *Periodontol* 25 (2001): 8–20.

Kinane D. F., I. G. Chestnutt. "Smoking and periodontal disease." *Crit Rev Oral Biol Med* 11 (2000): 356–365.

Kucukcoskun, Meric, Ulku Baser, Gorkem Oztekin, Esen Kiyan, Funda Yalcin. "Initial periodontal treatment for prevention of Chronic Obstructive pulmonary disease exacerbations." *Journal of Periodontology* 84(7) (July 2013): 863-70.

Laine, M.A. "Effect of pregnancy on periodontal and dental health." *Acta Odontol Scand.* 60(5) (2002): 257–264.

Libby, Peter, Paul M. Ridker. "Inflammation and atherosclerosis: Role of C-reactive protein in risk assessment." *Am J Med* 116 (Suppl. 6A) (2004): 9S–16S.

Libby, Peter, Paul M. Ridker, and Attilio Maseri. "Inflammation and Atherosclerosis." *Circulation* 05 (2002): 1135-1143, https://www.ahajournals.org/doi/full/10.1161/hc0902.104353.

Lieff, Susan, Kim A. Boggess, Amy P. Murtha, Heather Jared, Phoebus N. Madianos, Kevin Moss, James Beck, Steven

Offenbacher. "The oral conditions and pregnancy study: Periodontal status of a cohort of pregnant women." *J Periodontol*. 75(1) (Jan 2004): 116-26.

Lockhart, P.B. "The risk for endocarditis in dental practice." *Periodontol* 23 (2000): 127–135.

Loe, Harald. "Experimental gingivitis in man." *Journal of Periodontology*, 36.3 (1965): 177-187.

Loe, H., J. Silness. "Periodontal disease during pregnancy I. Prevalence and severity." *Acta Odontol Scand*. 21 (1963 Dec): 533-51.

Loos, B.G. "Systemic markers of inflammation in periodontitis." *J Periodontol* 76(Suppl. 11) (2005): 2106–2115.

Lösche, W., F. Karapetow, A. Pohl, C. Pohl, T. Kocher. "Plasma lipid, and glucose levels in patients with destructive periodontal disease." *J Clin Periodontol* 27(8) (2000): 537–541.

Manwell, M.A., L.S. Miller, D. Newbold, et al. "The relationship between reduction in periodontal inflammation and diabetes control: A report of 9 cases." *J Periodontol* (1992): 63: 843–848.

Mealey, Brian, Thomas Oates. "Diabetes Mellitus and Periodontal disease." *Journal of Periodontology* 77(8) (2006): 1289-1303.

Meisel, P., B. Holtfreter, H. Völzke, T. Kocher. "Sex differences of tooth loss and obesity on systemic markers of inflammation." *J Dent Res* 93 (2014): 774-779.

Meurman, J.H. "Oral microbiota and cancer." *J Oral Microbiol* 2 (2010): 1-10.

Michaud, D.S., K.T. Kelsey, E. Papathanasiou, C.A. Genco, E. Giovannucci. "Periodontal disease and risk of all cancers among male never smokers: An updated analysis of the health professional's follow-up study." *Ann Oncol* 27 (2016): 941–947.

Minihane, Anne M., Sophie Vinoy, Wendy R. Russell, Athanasia Baka, Helen M. Roche, Kieran M. Tuohy, Jessica L. Teeling, et al.

"Low-grade inflammation, diet composition and health: current research evidence and its translation." *The British Journal of Nutrition* 114.7 (2015): 999–1012, https://www.ncbi.nlm.nih.gov/pmc/articles/PMC4579563/.

Moludi, Jalal, Vahid Maleki, Hamed Jafari-Vayghyan, Elnaz Vaghef-Mehrabany, Mohammad Alizadeh. "Metabolic endotoxemia and cardiovascular disease: A systematic review about potential roles of prebiotics and probiotics." *Clinical Exp Pharmacol Physiol* 47(6) (2020): 927-939.

Montebugnoli, L., D. Servidio, R. A. Miaton, C. Prati, P. Tricoci, C. Melloni, G. Melandri. "Periodontal health improves systemic inflammatory and haemostatic status in subjects with coronary heart disease." *J Clin Periodontol* 32 (2005): 188–192.

Mougeot, J.C., C.B. Stevens, B.J. Paster, M.T. Brennan, P.B. Lockhart, F.K. Mougeot. "Porphyromonas Gingivalis is the most abundant species detected in coronary and femoral arteries." *J Oral Microbiol.* 9 (2017): 1281562.

Nabers, Claude. "Tooth loss in 1535 treated periodontal patients." *Journal of Periodontology* 59.5 (1988): 297-300.

Nascimento, G.G., K.G. Peres, M.N. Mittinty, et al. "Obesity and periodontal outcomes: a population-based cohort study in Brazil." *J Periodontol.* 88 (2017): 50-58.

Nascimento, Gustavo G., Fábio R. M. Leite, Karen G. Peres, Flávio F. Demarco, Marcos B. Corrêa, Marco A. Peres. "Metabolic syndrome and periodontitis: A structural equation modeling approach." *J Periodontol.* 90(6) (2019 Jun): 655-662.

Nelson, Robert G., Marc Shlossman, Lynn M. Budding, David J. Pettitt, Mohammed F. Saad, Robert J. Genco, and William C. Knowler. "Periodontal disease and NIDDM in Pima Indians." *Diabetes Care* 13(8) (1990): 836–840. http://dx.doi.org/10.2337/diacare.13.8.836.

Noack, B., R. J. Genco, M. Trevisan, S. Grossi, J. J. Zambon, E. De Nardin. "Periodontal infections contribute to elevated systemic C-reactive protein level." *J Periodontol.* 72 (2001): 1221–1227.

Noce, Annalisa, Giulia Marrone, Francesca Di Daniele, Eleonora Ottaviani, Georgia Wilson Jones, Roberta Bernini, Annalisa Romani, Valentina Rovella. "Impact of Gut Microbiota Composition on the Onset and Progression of Chronic Non-Communicable Diseases." *Nutrients* 11(5) (May 2019): 1073.

Offenbacher, Steven, James D. Beck, Heather L. Jared, Sally M. Mauriello, Luisto C. Mendoza, David J. Couper, Dawn D. Stewart, et al. "Effect of periodontal therapy on rate of preterm delivery: A randomized controlled trial." *Obstet Gynocol.* 114(3) (2009 Sep): 551–559.

Offenbacher, S., V. Katz, G. Fertik, J. Collins, D. Boyd, G. Maynor, R. McKaig, J. Beck. "Periodontal disease as a risk factor for preterm low birth weight." *J. Periodontology* 67(10 Suppl) (1996): 1103-13.

Olsen, I. "From the Acta prize lecture 2014: the periodontal-systemic connection seen from a microbiological standpoint." *Acta Odontol Scand.* 73(8) (2015): 563–5.

Olsen, Ingar, Steven D, Hicks. "Oral microbiota and autism spectrum disorder (ASD)." *J Oral Microbiol.* 12(1) (2019 Dec): 1702806.

Olsen, I., S.K. Singhrao. "Can oral infection be a risk factor for Alzheimer's disease?" *J Oral Microbiol.* 7 (2015): 29143.

Olsen, Ingar, Martin A. Taubman, Sim K. Singhrao. "Porphyromonas Gingivalis suppresses adaptive immunity in periodontitis, atherosclerosis, and Alzheimer›s disease." *J Oral Microbiol.* 8 (Nov 2016): 33029.

Olsen, Ingar, Kazuhisa Yamazaki. "Can oral bacteria affect the microbiome of the gut?" *J. Oral Microbio* 11(1) (2019): 1586422.

Olsen, I., Ö Yilmaz. "Possible role of *Porphyromonas Gingivalis* in orodigestive cancers." *J. Oral Microbio.* 11 (2018): 1563410.

Palmer, Richard M., Ron F. Wilson, Adam S. Hasan, David A. Scott. "Mechanisms of action of environmental factors – Tobacco smoking." *J Clin Periodontol* 32 (Suppl. 6) (2005): 180–195.

Pereira, P.A.B., V.T.E Aho, L. Paulin, et al. "Oral and nasal microbiota in Parkinson's disease." *Parkinsonism Relat Disord.* 38 (2017): 61-67.

Peter, Kalpak Prafulla, Bhumika Ramchandra Mute, Satish Shripad Doiphode, Suhas Jagannath Bardapurkar, Mangala Sonawani Borkar, Dhananjay Vasant Raje. "Association between periodontal disease and chronic obstructive pulmonary disease: A reality or just a dogma?" *J Periodontol* 84(12) (2013): 1717–1723.

Pink, C., T. Kocher, P. Meisel, et al. "Longitudinal effects of systemic inflammation markers on periodontitis." *J Clin Periodontol* 42 (2015): 988–997.

Pischon, N., N. Heng, J.P. Bernimoulin, B.M. Kleber, S.N. Willich, T. Pischon. "Obesity, inflammation, and periodontal disease." *J Dent Res* 86 (2007): 400-409.

Pitiphat, Waranuch, Kaumudi J. Joshipura, Janet W. Rich-Edwards, Paige L. Williams, Chester W. Douglass. Matthew W. Gillman. "Periodontitis and Plasma C-Reactive Protein During Pregnancy." *Journal of Periodontology* 77(5) (2006): 821–825.

Poole, S., S.K. Singhrao, L. Kesavalu, M.A. Curtis, S. Crean. "Determining the presence of periodontopathic virulence factors in short-term postmortem Alzheimer's disease brain tissue." *J Alzheimers Dis.* 36 (2013): 665-677.

Prado, G. "Not flossing could have dire health consequences." *Business Insider*, 2015, June 16. Retrieved December 22, 2020, from https://www.businessinsider.com/the-links-between-flossing-and-longevity-2015-6.

Pushalkar, Smruti, Xiaojie Ji, Yihong Li, Cherry Estilo, Ramanathan Yegnanarayana, Bhuvanesh Singh, Xin Li, Deepak Saxena. "Comparison of oral microbiota in tumor and non-tumor tissues of patients with oral squamous cell carcinoma." *BMC Microbiol* 12 (2012): 144.

Pussinen, Pirkko, Matti Jauhianen, Tiina Vilkuna-Rautiainen. "Periodontitis decreases the antiatherogenic potency of high density lipoprotein." *J Lipid Res.* 45 (2004): 139–147.

Ruiz, D.R., G.A. Romito, S.A. Dib. "Periodontal disease in gestational and type 1 diabetes mellitus pregnant women." *Oral Dis* 17 (2011): 515–521.

Saito, T., Y. Shimazaki. "Metabolic disorders related to obesity and periodontal disease." *Periodontol 2000* 43 (2007): 254-266.

Salazar, C.R., J.Sun, Y. Li, et al. "Association between selected oral pathogens and gastric precancerous lesions." *PLoS One* 8 (2013): e51604.

Saremi, Aramesh, Robert G. Nelson, Marshall Tulloch-Reid, Robert L. Hanson, Maurice L. Sievers, George W. Taylor, Marc Shlossman, et al. "Periodontal disease and mortality in type 2 diabetes." *Diabetes Care* 28(1) (2005): 27–32.

Sastrowijoto, S.H., P. Hillemans, T. J. van Steenbergen, L. Abraham-Inpijn, J. de Graaff. "Periodontal condition and microbiology of healthy and diseased periodontal pockets in type 1 diabetes mellitus patients." *J Clin Periodontol.* 16(5) (1989): 316–322.

Sato, Keisuke, Naoki Takahashi, Tamotsu Kato, Yumi Matsuda, Mai Yokoji, Miki Yamada, Takako Nakajima. "Aggravation of collagen-induced arthritis by orally administered *Porphyromonas Gingivalis* through modulation of the gut microbiota and gut immune system." *Nature Sci Rep.* 7(1) (2017): 6955.

Saygun, I., N. Nizam, I. Keskiner, V. Bal, A. Kubar, C. Açıkel, M. Serdar, J. Slots. "Salivary infectious agents and periodontal disease status." *J Periodontal Res.* 46(2) (2011): 235–239.

Scannapieco, F.A. "Role of oral bacteria in respiratory infection." *J Periodontol* 70 (1999): 793–802.

Scannapieco, Frank A., Renee B. Bush, Susanna Paju. "Associations between periodontal disease and risk for atherosclerosis, cardiovascular disease and stroke. A systematic review." *Ann Periodontol.* 8(1) (2003 Dec): 38-53, doi: 10.1902/annals.2003.8.1.38.

Scannapieco, F.A., A.W. Ho. "Potential associations between chronic respiratory disease and periodontal disease: Analysis of National Health and Nutrition Examination Survey III." *J Periodontol* 72(1) (2001): 50–56.

Scannapieco, F.A., G.D. Papandonatos, R.G. Dunford. "Associations between oral conditions and respiratory disease in a national sample survey population." *Ann Periodontol* 3(1) (1998): 251–256.

Scannapieco, F.A., B. Wang, H.J. Shiau. "Oral bacteria and respiratory infection: Effects on respiratory pathogen adhesion and epithelial cell proinflammatory cytokine production." *Ann Periodontol* 6(1) (2001): 78–86.

Schenkein, Harvey A., and Bruno G. Loos. "Inflammatory mechanisms linking periodontal diseases to cardiovascular disease." *Journal of Periodontology* 84(40) (April 2013): S51–S69.

Seedorf, Henning, Nicholas W. Griffin, Vanessa K. Ridaura, Alejandro Reyes, Jiye Cheng, Federico E. Rey, Michelle I. Smith. "Bacteria from diverse habitats colonize and compete in the mouse gut." *Cell* 159(2) (2014): 253–266.

Sen, Souvik, Kevin Moss, Lauren D. Giamberardino, Thiago Morelli, Wayne D. Rosamond, Rebecca F. Gottesman, James Beck, and Steven Offenbacher. "Periodontal disease, regular dental care use and incident ischemic stroke." *Stroke* 49 (2018): 355–362.

Seymour, G. J., P. J. Ford, M. P. Cullinan, S. Leishman, K. Yamazaki. "Relationship between periodontal infections and systemic disease." *Clin Microbiol Infect* 13 Suppl 4 (2007): 3–10.

Siegel, R., J. Ma, Z. Zou, A. Jemal. "Cancer statistics, 2014." *CA Cancer J Clin* 64 (2014): 9-29.

Srikantha, P., M.H. Mohajeri. "The possible role of the microbiota-gut-brain-axis in autism spectrum disorder." *Int J Mol Sci.* 20(9) (2019) pii: E2115.

Sun, Jinghua, Min Zhou, Christian R. Salazar, Rosemary Hays, Sukhleen Bedi, Yu Chen, Yihong Li. "Chronic Periodontal Disease, Periodontal Pathogen Colonization, and Increased Risk of Precancerous Gastric Lesions." *J Periodontol.* 88(11) (2017 Nov): 1124-1134.

Suvan, J., F. D'Aiuto, D.R. Moles, A. Petrie, N. Donos. "Association between overweight/obesity and periodontitis in adults. A systematic review." *Obes Rev* 12 (2011): e381-e404.

Taylor, G. W., B. A. Burt, M. P. Becker, R. J. Genco, M. Shlossman, W. C. Knowler, D. J. Pettitt. "Severe periodontitis and risk for poor glycemic control in patients with non-insulin-dependent diabetes mellitus." *J Periodontol.* 67(10 Suppl) (1996 Oct): 1085-93, doi: 10.1902/jop.1996.67.10s.1085.

Taylor, G.W., W.J. Loesche, M.S. Terpenning. "Impact of oral diseases on systemic health in the elderly: Diabetes mellitus and aspiration pneumonia." *J Public Health Dent* 60(4) (2000): 313-320.

Terpenning, M.S. "The relationship between infections and chronic respiratory diseases: An overview." *Ann Periodontol* 6(1) (2001): 66–70.

Torre, L.A., R.L. Siegel, E.M. Ward, A. Jemal. "Global cancer incidence and mortality rates and trends – An update." *Cancer Epidemiol Biomarkers Prev* 25 (2016):16–27.

"Understanding Inflammation." *Harvard Health Publishing.* Retrieved December 22, 2020. https://www.health.harvard.edu/staying-healthy/understanding-inflammation.

US Department of Health and Human Services. "2014 Surgeon General's Report: The Health Consequences of Smoking — 50 Years of Progress." Retrieved November 13, 2020. https://www.

cdc.gov/tobacco/data_statistics/sgr/50th-anniversary/index.htm#report.

van Winkelhoff, A. J., C. J. Bosch-Tijhof, E. G. Winkel, W. A. van der Reijden. "Smoking affects the subgingival microflora in periodontitis." *J Periodontol* 72(5) (2001): 666–671.

Vergnes J.N., M. Sixou. "Preterm low birth weight and maternal periodontal status: A meta-analysis." *Am J Obstet Gynecol* 196(2) (2007): 135.e1–7.

von Troil-Lindén, B., H. Torkko, S. Alaluusua, H. Jousimies-Somer, S. Asikainen. "Salivary levels of suspected periodontal pathogens in relation to periodontal status and treatment." *J Dent Res*. 74(11) (1995): 1789–1795.

Vuong, H.E., J.M. Yano, T.C. Fung, et al. "The microbiome and host behavior." *Annu Rev Neurosci*. 40 (2017): 21-49.

Wang, M., J. Zhou, F. He, et al. "Alteration of gut microbiota-associated epitopes in children with autism spectrum disorders." *Brain Behav Immun*. 75 (2019): 192–199.

Warnakulasuriya, Saman, Thomas Dietrich, Michael M Bornstein, Elías Casals Peidró, Philip M Preshaw, Clemens Walter, Jan L Wennström, Jan Bergström. "Oral health risks of tobacco use and effects of cessation." *Int Dent J.* 60 (2010) :7–30.

Watanabe, K., Y.D. Cho. "Periodontal disease and metabolic syndrome: A qualitative critical review of their association." *Arch Oral Biol* 59 (2014): 855-870.

Weigang, L.,P. Girvan, P. Ingmudsen, R. Verrett, J. Schoolfield, B. Mealey. "Investigating the Association between onstructive sleep apnea and periodontitis." *J. Periodontol* 86(2) (2015).

Woelber, Johan P., Maximilian Gärtner, Lilian Breuninger, Annette Anderson, Daniel König, Elmar Hellwig, Ali Al-Ahmad, Kirstin Vach, Andreas Dötsch, Petra Ratka-Krüger, Christian Tennert. "The influence of an anti-inflammatory diet on gingivitis. A randomized controlled trial." *J. of Clinical Periodontology* 46(4) (Apr. 2019): 481-490.

World Health Organization. "Obesity: Preventing and Managing the Global Epidemic: Report of a WHO Consultation." *WHO Tech.* (2000) Rep. Ser. 894. Geneva.

Xiong, X., L. D. Saunders, F. L. Wang, N. N. Demianczuk. "Gestational diabetes mellitus: Prevalence, risk factors, maternal and infant outcomes." *Int J Gynaecol Obstet* 75(3) (2001): 221–228.

Xiong, Xu, Karen E. Elkind-Hirsch, Sotirios Vastardis, Robert L. Delarosa, Gabriella Pridjian, Pierre Buekens. "Periodontal disease is associated with gestational diabetes mellitus: A case-control study." *J Periodontol* 80 (2009): 1742–1749.

Young, T., M. Palta, J. Dempsey, J. Skatrud, S. Weber, S. Badr. "The occurrence of sleep-disordered breathing among middle-aged adults." *N Engl J Med*. 328(17) (1993):1230-5. doi: 10.1056/NEJM199304293281704. PMID: 8464434.

Zelkha, S.A., R.W. Freilich, S. Amar. "Periodontal innate immune mechanisms relevant to atherosclerosis and obesity." *Periodontol 2000* 54 (2010): 207-221.

Lightning Source UK Ltd.
Milton Keynes UK
UKHW022144260922
409472UK00007B/1024